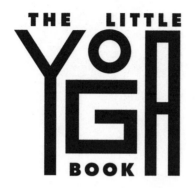

THE LITTLE
YOGA
BOOK

THE LITTLE
YOGA
BOOK

ERIKA DILLMAN

WARNER BOOKS

A Time Warner Company

Neither these yoga exercises and programs nor any other exercise program should be followed without first consulting a health care professional. If you have any special conditions requiring attention, you should consult with your health care professional regularly regarding possible modification of the program contained in this book.

Warner Books, Inc., 1271 Avenue of the Americas, New York, NY 10020
Visit our Web site at http://warnerbooks.com

 A Time Warner Company

Printed in the United States of America
First Printing: January 1999
10 9 8 7

Library of Congress Cataloging-in-Publication Data

Dillman, Erika.
    The little yoga book
       p. cm.
    ISBN 0-446-67392-7
    1. Yoga.
  BL1238.52.D55   1999
  613.7'046—dc21   98-21254
                                                         CIP

Book design and text composition by L&G McRee
Illustrations beginning on page 42 by Georg Brewer
Cover design by Rachel McClain

ATTENTION: SCHOOLS AND CORPORATIONS
WARNER books are available at quantity discounts with bulk purchase for educational, business, or sales promotional use. For information, please write to: SPECIAL SALES DEPARTMENT, WARNER BOOKS, 1271 AVENUE OF THE AMERICAS, NEW YORK, N.Y. 10020

For my grandmother
Hanna Anderson

Acknowledgments

I would like to thank the following people for their contributions to *The Little Yoga Book*:

Denise Andersen for teaching me the importance of alignment.

My agent, Anne Depue, for believing in my book.

My friends for their encouragement and support.

My yoga teacher, Suzanne Guttridge, for her wisdom and fun yoga. May her spirit live on in these pages.

Cornelia Bremer Smith, Debby Heath, Laura Prindiville, Jane Whitlock, Jonathan Pettigrew, and Rob White for test driving the pose instructions.

Sarah Schultz, Emily Stevens, and Sandi Sonnenfeld for their editorial suggestions.

Contents

Welcome to
The Little Yoga Book

My goal in writing this book is to demystify yoga for people who are looking for a simple, nonthreatening introduction to this ancient health practice. When I first discovered yoga, I was overwhelmed by all of the different philosophies and disciplines which accompanied the exercise. I just wanted to learn how to relax and to improve my posture. That is why I have focused here primarily on the physical aspects of yoga.

The Little Yoga Book is a portable companion, a guide to inspire and structure your practice. I have included forty-two of my favorite poses, as well as several breathing exercises, that are commonly taught in beginning- and intermediate-level yoga classes.

The main purpose behind this "little" book is to help make yoga manageable and accessible to a variety of people. I have written all of the exercises in the same easy-to-follow format for practicing alone or with a friend. The book is small so that you can take it with you wherever you go—to class, to work, or on vacation.

If you've never done yoga before, I recommend taking some classes because the best way to learn yoga is from a good teacher. If you have studied yoga, or are just starting to learn about it, you'll recognize a lot of the poses here, and I hope they will become part of your daily routine.

Enjoy.

Introduction

LOSING BALANCE

Before I began studying yoga almost four years ago, I was a runner. I started running in sixth grade and it quickly became a vital part of my life. Running centered me, cleared my head of stress and negativity, boosted my confidence, and strengthened my body. The high from the endorphins my body produced during my runs was the best part. Sometimes I felt that I went into another state of being during a run, a feeling to which I became addicted.

"No Pain, No Gain" seemed like a perfectly legitimate motto to me, so I pushed my body to run every day whether it was −10°F or 95°F outside, whether I was healthy or ill. I ran through fatigue, mononucleosis, pneumonia, strained muscles, torn fascia, and fractured bones. When I was forced to take off time to heal an injury, I just transferred the same intensity to swimming. In fact, I applied the same intensity to most things I did.

Eventually, my body rebelled and I began having health problems that stopped me from running or doing any exercise. An acute case of bronchitis had left me with inflamed lungs, asthma, and chest pains. My lungs felt like they were made out of thick, scratchy wool that rubbed against the inside of my chest, making breathing painful and leaving me perpetually exhausted.

My body felt like it was falling apart, and my immune system was in overdrive. Every substance I came into contact with, every movement I made, seemed to make me ill. I struggled to get through each day, overwhelmed by dizziness, chest pains, nausea, and numbness in my hands, arms, and face so severe that I often became disoriented and faint. Finally, a little over a year after my health had progressively deteriorated, I was diagnosed with Chronic Fatigue Immune Dysfunction Syndrome (CFIDS). When my doctors couldn't cure me, I was devastated. I didn't know how to get my health back, and nothing I tried seemed to make me feel better.

During this time I began drawing cartoons of my life to express my anger, sadness, and utter frustration at living with a chronic illness. Unable to live the physical existence that I was used to, I felt helpless, lost, and completely disconnected from my body and my identity. If I couldn't run, I didn't know how to make myself feel good mentally or physically.

I was sick of writing about my problems in my journal, confiding in friends and family, and constantly trying to explain an illness that many people didn't believe in and nobody understood. In one of my first pictures, *Erika Nervosa*, tears arc from my eyes and thought bubbles, bursting with frantic stress and worry, crash into each other over my head. Images of every possible stressor crowd in around me: my illness, my job, my husband, my family, my doctors, environmental disasters, and my dwindling MCI calling circle.

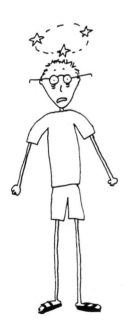

In another drawing I'm huddled in the corner of the page, cowering, exhausted, dizzy, with dark circles under my eyes. Moving in to attack me from every direction are human-sized dust mites, bumble bees, cats, dogs, and gigantic flowers—all of them bearing a frowning, evil version of my husband's normally cheerful face.

I didn't think to analyze what the drawings meant for several months. Apparently, my body's intelligence knew what was happening to me, but I couldn't understand it or fix it. When I eventually did look at the pictures as something other than a humorous attempt to deflect how low I felt, it was so obvious. The first picture was my mind out of balance, and the second picture was my body out of balance. All of the animal, bug, and plant aggressors represented the many substances which battered my malfunctioning immune system, leaving me weak and debilitated.

I suppose these drawings were my first steps in mind-body awareness because I soon realized that I had to find a way to regain my equilibrium.

People suggested all sorts of cures for CFIDS: acupuncture, blue-green algae, Chinese herbs—all of which I did try eventually. But the alternative treatments were too much like regular medicine; they required me to take pills, go to offices for treatments, and rely on other people to change my health.

I needed something deeper that would calm me down and help me reconnect with my body. More important, I wanted to do something physical, something that came from within me, so that I could regain confidence in myself and take charge of my health.

Desperate to get my old body back and learn how to breathe again, I turned to yoga.

1/Discovering Yoga

THE YOGA DICTATOR

I had done some yoga breathing once when a yoga teacher came to my office to conduct a relaxation workshop. The breathing exercises had helped my lungs and my head feel better, although I felt a little funny lying on the floor making breathing noises in front of my co-workers. Something that the teacher said had stuck with me, even though I didn't fully believe it. She said that yoga helped balance and unite mind and body.

Curious to find out more and propelled by desperation, I signed up for my first yoga class, despite a lingering skepticism. Breathing exercises in my office were one thing, but I was sort of a jock. I had never appreciated the value of an exercise that didn't involve sweat, pain, and competition. And weren't yoga people kind of weird? I wasn't too sure about meeting them on their own turf.

I associated yoga with a murky, mystical, other-worldly aura. I imagined dark rooms filled with patchouli incense and rows of thin, ascetic men and women sitting in the lotus position, chanting in trance-like unison. I couldn't shake from my mind the pictures I'd seen in yoga books of gaunt, solemn men, wearing what looked like giant diapers, with one leg wrapped around their necks, and cold, expressionless women in Jack LaLanne–style polyester unitards nonchalantly twisting, bending, and lifting themselves into torturous positions.

These images intimidated me because I knew that MY body could never do that, but also because I didn't feel any energy or joy from the pictures. They were too serious and nobody seemed to be having any fun. I thought that they must all belong to a secret club where everyone was miserable. That was the price you had to pay for enlightenment.

Unfortunately, my worst suspicions were confirmed when I attended my first yoga class. I was pretty nervous about being there because I didn't like putting myself into unfamiliar physical situations when I was so out of shape. I didn't know the rituals, the lingo, the protocol. And I had long before lost all confidence in my frail body.

The teacher, a brisk, short, hard-eyed woman in a tight aqua-blue unitard, came in, took my money (scolded me for paying with a check), and sent me to the other side of the room. As other people filed in and took their spaces on the floor, I started to feel dreadful. Once the class began I had no idea what the teacher was doing or how to breathe.

I struggled with every pose, feeling weak, tired, and foolish. At one point, the teacher marched over to me, grabbed my head and pulled it down into her face, rubbing my forehead with her thick, strong thumbs, commanding, "You cannot do yoga with a grimace! Open your third eye." I was dying. I'd tried so hard to blend in and not make a spectacle of myself, and there I was with everyone looking at me and my third eye refusing to cooperate. I was determined to make it through the class, though, and I stuck with it, trying not to grimace as I twisted and contorted my scrawny, inflexible body.

Occasionally, the yoga dictator came over and yanked the hair on top of my head to remind me to stand up straight. Then, just when I was starting to feel like she'd forgotten about me, she called me to the front of the room to help her demonstrate a pose for the class. She stood bolt upright and started tightening and flexing her buttock muscles and rotating her ankles in some bizarre pose. Then she grabbed my hands, placed them on her butt and told me to hold on to her, then slide my hands down her legs to her ankles, so I could feel what her muscles were doing.

Okay. I'm from the Midwest; we don't touch other peoples' butts. Not for any reason. And we certainly don't do it in front of a room full of mirrors and people dressed in black leotards. I was mortified. As soon as class was over, I fled, traumatized (but with better posture). I never went back, and it took an entire year for me to try yoga again.

I realized later that I had let my misconceptions about yoga get to me, and my pride keep me from looking for another class. The fact that the yoga dictator has classes to teach means that some people enjoy and thrive under a strict, disciplined format, but that style didn't work for me.

Before my illness I had always jumped into new situations, able to start in the middle, but that wasn't who I was when I was sick. I needed a different approach. I had to start at the beginning, and I needed basic instructions, patience (from myself and from my teacher), and a minimum of jargon about third eyes.

4

I Start Bending

My second attempt at yoga came a year later, after nearly two years of illness. My condition had become worse, and I'd been forced to quit my job. I spent six months doing nothing but sleeping and worrying that I was dying. Too exhausted and disoriented to drive a car, read, or talk on the phone, I spent most of my days and nights lying on the couch, staring vacantly at the TV. Despite sleeping twelve to fourteen hours a night, taking a two-hour nap after breakfast, and another nap after lunch, I was still too exhausted most days even to shower. My formerly strong, athletic body became weak, atrophied, and emaciated. I had no energy, and I was deeply depressed.

After another few months, anxious to get moving again, I began taking short five-minute walks to the grocery store a couple of times a week. One day I saw a bright pink flyer on the store bulletin board that advertised "FUN Yoga." After talking with the teacher on the phone, I felt relieved. She seemed to understand my situation, and her kind voice put me at ease. The class sounded like just what I needed to get started: breathing exercises and stretching and flexibility poses—all at my own pace. This time it was going to be different. I was determined to reconnect with my body, and I knew that if I could do that I could also ease the tension in my mind.

I was still a bit self-conscious when I arrived at class a few days later, but I soon felt that I was in the right place. There were only a handful of people sitting and talking on the floor in a small, dark room, and they all looked pretty normal. No fancy unitards, no mirrors, no solemn faces, just ordinary people in baggy sweats and T-shirts. As we went around the room introducing ourselves, I realized that I wasn't the only beginner or the only person with health problems.

The class lasted an hour, but I ran out of steam after five minutes. I was so frail; every movement sent me into a coughing, choking fit. I spent the rest of the class exhausted and dizzy, resting on my blanket and trying to stay awake.

Within about four months, three women and myself had become the core group of "regulars." Because the class was small we each received a lot of personal attention, which helped us gain confidence in learning the poses, and we became friends. We lingered after class to talk about our respective health rituals and swap phone numbers for naturopaths, acupuncturists, and massage therapists. I looked forward to the class every week because it was the one time I got out of the house and had some fun.

Unlike in the yoga dictator's class, we laughed as we attempted to twist, bend, and stretch our unwilling bodies into alignment. We whined about doing difficult poses (I used to ask, "Can't we do the yoga of lying down?"), and we often joked that someone should put *us*, with all of our giggling and imperfections, in a yoga video called "Yoga for Real People."

By this time I had worked up to doing fifteen minutes of yoga each class before I had to rest, and it took another two or three months before I could last for thirty minutes. Finally, after nine months, my lungs became less sensitive, my breathing improved, and I noticed that I was able to do several of the poses without collapsing.

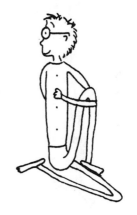

During this period, I continued to draw my cartoons, and they slowly changed. I no longer drew myself as a cowering victim, although I still sometimes drew myself as a weak, exhausted skinny person. More often, I drew the me I *wanted* to be: smiling, active, energetic. I started drawing myself doing yoga, socializing with friends, and working at my desk, hoping that my body would someday catch up with my cartoon self.

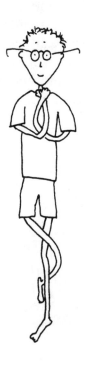

I also drew because I found in my daily practice that I couldn't always remember the poses I had learned in class. Once I saw a picture, though, my body remembered exactly what to do. The more poses I learned, the more pictures I drew. After time, my yoga practice and my drawing both improved and began to enhance each other.

When I was drawing I started to see new possibilities in how I approached the poses that I was struggling to master in class. And when I was learning a new pose in class, I visualized my cartoon self in the pose so that I would be able to draw it later. This process helped me take a few more steps toward mind-body awareness.

After a year, I was able to last through an entire class, sitting out only a few poses, and practicing at home a couple of days a week for about ten minutes a session. Now, four years later, I attend an hour-long yoga class once a week that emphasizes strength and stamina poses, I practice at home for ten to twenty minutes four or five days a week, and I take my yoga mat with me whenever I travel.

As my yoga practice has improved, my drawings have become more active, more hopeful, and more energized. I draw myself running, practicing more difficult yoga poses, and even swinging upside down on a trapeze.

I am still struggling with my illness. Yoga hasn't cured me of CFIDS, but it has become an important part of my life. It helps me wake up in the morning, get the kinks out of my back after I've been working on my computer, and stay sane until I can run again. I often use yoga breathing exercises during the day to relax and clear my mind when my life gets too hectic.

I've been surprised to learn that many of the physical and mental benefits I got from running, such as stress relief, physical strength, concentration, and a general feeling of well-being, I now get from yoga. I'm much more flexible than

I ever was as a runner, which I know will help prevent injuries when I am able to be more active. Most important, yoga has helped me understand the value of balance, patience, and slowing down.

2/What Is Yoga?

STRETCH, BREATHE, LIVE

There is no big, mystical secret to yoga. It is not a religion, although some people use yoga to achieve spiritual enlightenment. It is not calisthenics, although it does exercise, stretch, and strengthen the body. Yoga is a system of physical and mental exercises designed thousands of years ago to balance and unite mind, body, and spirit.

There are many different types of yoga, each with its own philosophies and practices. Some yogas are meditative and focused on spiritual centeredness, others are more physical and based on poses, or exercises, called asanas. While many schools of yoga share common qualities, they also vary in focus and practice. For example, one ancient yoga text refers to hundreds of thousands of different yoga poses, while other sources, in-

11

cluding modern interpretations of ancient texts, recommend that of the many yoga poses in existence, only a few dozen to a few hundred be used in practice.

To keep this book simple, I will be focusing primarily on the physical aspects of yoga (and the belief that there are hundreds, if not thousands, of yoga poses). If you want to pursue a deeper spiritual study of yoga, check your library for a list of yoga books covering that topic, or look for a yoga class that is more spiritually oriented. There are also quite a few yoga web sites now on the Internet. (Also, please note that while there are excellent yoga teachers of both genders, throughout the text I have referred to yoga teachers as "she" for simplicity and consistency.)

As you get more involved in your practice, you will quickly learn the beauty of yoga's simple and innate wisdom: that you can't separate mind, body, and spirit. By balancing your body, you'll learn to focus your mind, which in turn will improve your health and spiritual well-being. In other words, coordinating breathing exercises and concentration with the poses is in itself a form of meditation, so whether you come to yoga to learn how to relax or to get rid of the knots in your back, you'll be practicing and gaining benefits on many different levels.

The most common type of yoga taught in the United States is hatha yoga. Hatha, a Sanskrit word that means "sun" (ha) and "moon" (tha), represents the opposing energies in our bodies—hot and cold, male and female, positive and negative, yin and yang. Yoga, translated from *yuga*, the Sanskrit word for yoke, means union. Hatha yoga balances the mind and body through physical exercises (poses) and controlled breathing so that all of the body's energies can achieve equilibrium and function in harmony.

In the last several years yoga has become more popular because people are looking for a more holistic approach to health and exercise, and yoga, a dynamic exercise which is both relaxing and energizing, seems to have it all.

Yoga challenges mind and body, increases flexibility and stamina, builds strength, and improves balance and concentration. It also improves circulation, promotes relaxation, and benefits internal organs, glands, and muscles. Yoga can be done anywhere by people of all ages and abilities, and it doesn't require any special equipment. Most important, yoga teaches people how to be more in tune with their bodies, and how to be more aware of the mind-body connection.

As life becomes more complicated and hectic, and ailments

like Chronic Fatigue Immune Dysfunction Syndrome, Carpal Tunnel Syndrome, and back pain become more prevalent, even western-trained doctors are turning to yoga to treat their patients' illnesses and injuries.

The primary physical goal of yoga is to keep the spine flexible and strong. This makes a lot of sense when you remember that the spine is the body's supporting structure, as well as the center for nerves which supply the entire body. Many of us have poor posture, with hunched upper backs and swayed lower backs. Sitting at a desk all day, working on a computer, and just plain living in gravity all conspire to compact the spine.

Practicing yoga strengthens the body's major muscle groups to support the weight of your body, improving posture, or alignment. Correct alignment helps the body function more optimally, resulting in less pain, more freedom of movement, less fatigue, more flexibility, and more stamina. As my yoga teacher often reminds our class, "You're only as flexible as your spine!"

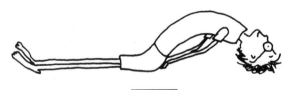

3/Before You Start

BASIC GUIDELINES

The best way to learn yoga is from an experienced yoga teacher. There are many types of yoga and many styles of teaching. You might have to try out a few classes until you find one that you like. Some classes focus on strengthening poses, others on breathing, or on flexibility. Look for a class that fits your needs. And look for a teacher who is patient, who is educated in how the body works and how each pose affects the body (and mind), and who takes time during class to give individual instruction.

Because there is no standard criteria among yoga schools, teaching certification varies. An important quality to look for in a teacher is her commitment to yoga as her primary health and/or spiritual practice. The teachers I have learned the most from have been teaching for over twenty years and are themselves lifetime yoga students, having studied with yoga masters (and continuing to study with them). Look for a teacher who not only has a deep knowledge of how yoga benefits mind and body but has integrated this knowledge into her lifestyle and daily habits.

A good teacher can make a huge difference in your practice. One of the most important ways that a teacher can help you is by adjusting your body when you practice each pose. With guidance, you'll start to learn what it feels like to be in alignment. As you learn more about yoga and become more aware of your alignment, you'll be able to transfer that posture to other activities in your life.

Once you begin taking a class, you can use this book to help you remember the poses for your home practice. If you've never done yoga before, I recommend that you wait to try any of the poses I've described until your teacher has shown you some of the basic yoga poses and how to coordinate your breathing with your movements.

Have patience. It takes many years of daily practice to become proficient in some yoga poses. If you practice regularly and take classes, you will begin to feel the benefits within a few months. Don't ever force your body into a pose, or make any movements that cause pain. Listen to your body. Take your time. Be gentle with yourself.

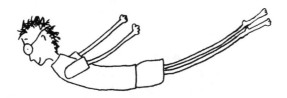

Feel free to adapt yoga to your own needs. If you have chronically tight hamstrings or sore computer arms or a stiff neck, ask your teacher which poses will help you feel better. Also, as you read through the instructions you might notice that there are poses you can't do because of existing injuries or deconditioning. Don't worry—all of the exercises in this book can be altered to help you get started. For example, if you can't kneel in a certain pose because it hurts your knees, then your teacher can show you another way to practice that pose (maybe sitting cross-legged on the floor) or show you another pose that you can do to gain similar benefits. As you develop greater mind-body awareness, you'll be able to make your own variations on the poses.

If you haven't been active for a long period of time, you might want to see your doctor before beginning any type of exercise program. If you are taking medication or have a medical condition or injury, especially heart problems, high blood pressure, back or neck problems, or if you are pregnant, make sure you tell your yoga teacher so that she can tell you if there are any poses that could aggravate your condition.

If you are pregnant, there are books available with instructions for practicing yoga during pregnancy, and many health clubs and community centers now offer prenatal yoga classes.

Drink a lot of water. Yoga is exercise, and the body needs to be replenished after exertion.

Wear comfortable clothing, remove shoes and socks, and practice yoga in a quiet, warm place on a mat or thick towel. Wait at least one to two hours after eating to begin practice. Unplug the phone so you can practice undisturbed.

Tips: • Hatha yoga is a gentle, flowing yoga, but that does not mean that you can't hurt yourself if you aren't careful. As with any form of exercise, you need to warm up, begin slowly, increase intensity slowly, and be aware of the messages your body sends you. During your practice, keep in mind the following general guidelines:

- *Watch Your Back!*
  With every pose, make sure that you are not straining your back, especially if you have back or neck problems. NEVER use jerky or fast movements. Ask your teacher to show you how to support your back during different poses.

- *Keep Your Balance!*
  Keep your body in balance by repeating the same pose for each side of the body and by practicing counterposes. For example, if you stretch your right arm in a pose, do the same stretch in your left arm. When practicing poses that arch the back, also practice poses that round the back. That way, the toning and strengthening benefits of yoga will align the body and promote fluidity and

energy. Don't be surprised if you can do a pose on one side of the body, but it's more difficult to do on the other side—that's normal.

- *Remember to Breathe!*
  Correct breathing increases yoga's benefits. It's easy to concentrate so hard on practicing the pose right that you forget to coordinate your movements with your breath. As a general rule, an inhaling breath accompanies an opening of the body, or a backward bend, and an exhaling breath accompanies a closing of the body, or a forward bend. With some poses, you will get into the pose first, then hold the pose for three to six breaths. Ask your teacher to show you how to use your breath to enter deeper into a pose.

- *Slow Down!*
  Yoga is never a competition. Your movements should be slow, fluid, and mindful, coordinated with the breath. Don't worry about doing the pose exactly like your teacher or like a picture in a

book. Relax, and practice the pose to your own limits. If you are in balance and breathing, you will gain benefits from your efforts.

- *Stand Tall!*
  The goal is to elongate the spine. One way to think of alignment is to visualize energy moving up the spine and out the top of your head. Whether you are practicing standing, lying down, sitting, or kneeling poses, strive to maintain correct alignment (which is described on page 43).

- *Have Fun!*
  Make yoga something you look forward to each day. Allow yourself to enjoy getting more in touch with your body. Buy yourself a nice yoga mat. Burn a candle or play classical music or a chanting monks CD before you practice to get into the mood. Draw pictures or write notes to help you remember difficult poses. Reward yourself with tea when you finish.

4/Breathing

THE IMPORTANCE OF CORRECT BREATHING

Breathing is a vital element of hatha yoga. Practicing yoga breathing, or pranayama, energizes and cleanses the body, serving as a perfect warm-up for practicing the poses. Pranayama is a Sanskrit word that means "breath control." By controlling your breath, you can calm and relax your mind and body.

Most people do not breathe efficiently, and as a result, use only a fraction of their lung capacity. Poor posture, tight clothing, and the hectic pace of life all interfere with breathing. When we are stressed or anxious, we breathe from our chests, talking rapid, shallow breaths, or worse, we hold our breath. Without sufficient oxygen, we become fatigued and lethargic.

For optimal health, breathing should be full and rhythmic, using the diaphragm and ribs to fill and empty the lungs. The goal of yoga breathing is to restore full function to the lungs, diaphragm, abdominal muscles, and ribs, which are all involved in correct breathing.

The complete change of air in the lungs increases oxygen levels in the body, which produces energy. The exhaling and inhaling breaths are equally important. The exhaling breath expels stale air, allowing the lungs to fill up fully with fresh air during inhalation.

In coordination with yoga poses, the breath unifies mind and body, balances opposing energies, and helps the body move deeper into each pose.

Learning how to control your breath can be a powerful health tool and stress buster. Breathing exercises increase your oxygen intake, improving circulation and the elimination of toxins; calm the mind and relax the body, improving concentration and mental clarity; and generally, increase energy levels.

YOGA BREATHING EXERCISES (PRANAYAMA)

The following pranayama exercises are common in yoga practice and will provide you with a good foundation from which to learn more. I selected these exercises because they were some of the first I learned and because they are relatively simple. As you master these exercises and learn more about yoga, ask your teacher about other pranayama exercises, such as the cleansing breath (Kapalabhati), the bellows breath (Bhastrika), the cooling breath (Sitali), and another cooling breath, sometimes called "hissing breath" (Sitkari).

If practicing any of these exercises makes you feel dizzy or uncomfortable, stop immediately and rest. These simple exercises can have a profound effect on the body, especially if you are not used to dealing with large volumes of oxygen. With practice, these exercises will improve your lung capacity and energy levels, as well as relax you.

Tips:
- Breathing exercises are usually done while sitting on heels with legs bent underneath you (see Thunderbolt pose, page 115) or sitting cross-legged on the floor. (Some exercises can be done lying down.)

- Yoga breathing is generally done through the nose.

- The goal of breathing exercises is to control the length and quality of the breath by slowing down your inhalations and exhalations.

- The exhaling breath should last as long as the inhaling breath. Making the exhaling breath last twice as long as the inhaling breath is even more beneficial. For example, if you inhale for three seconds, exhale for three to six seconds.

- Keep in mind the three main areas where you feel your breath as you inhale and exhale: the abdomen, or belly, which is below the navel; the diaphragm, which is above the navel; and the chest.

- Keep your belly relaxed in all of these exercises.

- Practice the breathing exercises in the order they appear.

Understanding abdominal and rib cage breathing is the first step in learning what it feels like to use different parts of your body to breathe correctly. The third exercise, Complete Breath, the ideal in yoga breathing, integrates these first two exercises.

ABDOMINAL BREATHING

Benefits: Relaxes mind and body, strengthens lungs, and massages internal organs.

Instructions:

1. Sit or lie completely still with hand placed on abdomen, just below navel.
2. Relax your mind and body so that you can feel the gentle rise and fall of the abdomen as your diaphragm naturally moves with your breathing.
3. Let the air move in and out of your body without effort.
4. As you inhale, you will feel your abdomen rise. As you exhale, you will feel your abdomen sink.
5. Practice this exercise for ten breaths. (One inhalation and one exhalation equals one breath.)

RIB CAGE BREATHING

Benefits: Relaxes mind and body, strengthens lungs.

Instructions:

1. Sit or lie completely still with hands placed on sides (ribs).
2. Gently contract abdomen so that when you inhale the breath fills the top part of your lungs.
3. Inhale into your rib cage. Do not pull the breath deep into your lungs, but keep it focused between your ribs.
4. Feel the ribs expand outward and the chest open as you breathe in. As you exhale, feel the ribs contract inward. Repeat five times.

COMPLETE BREATH

Benefits: The Complete Breath is full, deep, and slow, fully using the lungs and expanding the ribs and chest. With increased lung capacity, the body can more efficiently cleanse the blood.

Instructions:

1. Sit or lie completely still.
2. Exhale to clear the body of stale air.
3. Inhale, filling up the bottom of the lungs, the middle of the lungs, then slowly filling the chest.
4. Slowly exhale, emptying the lungs from top to bottom. Repeat five times.

Tip:
- As you inhale, you will feel your abdomen rise, then your diaphragm rise, and finally, your chest expand.

ALTERNATE NOSTRIL BREATHING

Benefits: Clears the nasal passages and calms the mind.

Instructions:

1. Sit on the floor in Thunderbolt pose or in cross-legged position.
2. Extend the thumb and ring and pinky fingers (holding these two fingers together) of right hand, leaving the other two fingers curled into palm.
3. Place thumb against right side of nose, sealing the right nostril closed. Inhale slowly and deeply through left nostril. Hold.
4. Then press ring and pinky fingers, keeping them together, against left side of nose, sealing the left nostril closed, and lift thumb from right side of nose, opening right nostril.
5. Exhale slowly and fully through right nostril. Hold.
6. Inhale slowly and deeply through right nostril, still holding left nostril shut. Hold.
7. Cover right nostril with thumb, releasing left nostril, and exhaling through left nostril.
8. Repeat sequence five times.

Tip: • If it is more comfortable, you can also do this breathing exercise using your thumb and middle finger, curling the ring and pinky fingers into palm, and resting your index finger along nose.

Tapping Chest Breath

Benefits: Stimulates lung cells, strengthens respiratory system.

Instructions:

1. Sit on the floor in Thunderbolt pose or in cross-legged position.
2. Inhale deeply, filling the lungs and expanding the chest. Hold.
3. With fingers of right hand, tap quickly and sharply all over chest.
4. Stop tapping, bending forward as you exhale through your mouth.
5. Relax. Repeat five times.

Bhramari Breath

Benefits: Vibrates and opens up the sinuses, clears the mind, and calms the nerves.

Instructions:

1. Sit on the floor in Thunderbolt pose or in cross-legged position.
2. Inhale, filling the lungs. Hold.
3. While exhaling slowly out of nostrils, hum an "m" sound and direct the vibration into facial area between the tops of the teeth and the eyes.
4. Contract ribs and squeeze area a few inches above navel to fully expel air. Repeat five times.

Ujjayi Breath

Benefits: Increases lung capacity, opens the chest, relaxes the nervous system, and increases oxygen in blood.

Instructions:

1. Sit on the floor in Thunderbolt pose or in cross-legged position.
2. Inhale slowly, keeping mouth closed and partially closing, or contracting, the back of your throat to slow down the breath. Hold for a few seconds.
3. Exhale, again partially closing or contracting at back of throat to slow down the breath. This breath will make a hoarse hiss-like sound like steam being released from a radiator. You will feel a slight pressure in the back of your nose as the air moves out of your nose during your exhaling breath.
4. Repeat five times.

Tips:
- Ujjayi is pronounced "U-ji."

- As you get better at Ujjayi breath, try to exhale for longer than you inhale.

- Ujjayi breath can also be done in coordination with poses for a further challenge.

5/How to Structure Your Practice

ELEMENTS OF PRACTICE

In order to maximize yoga's benefits, practice regularly and design an all-body routine that improves balance, flexibility, stamina, and strength. A well-rounded practice includes the following types of poses: abdominal strengtheners, backward and forward bends, balancing, spinal twists, and poses that stretch and strengthen the legs, hips, arms, shoulders, neck, and back.

When I practice yoga at home, I tend to do my favorite poses every day, in no specific order. Once a week I attend a class so that I can break out of my rut and try new poses. I find that the poses I avoid practicing at home because they are too challenging are exactly the exercises my body most needs to do.

Begin your yoga practice with a few minutes of breathing exercises (pages 24–33) and warm-up exercises (pages 63–74). In *The Complete Yoga Book* by James Hewitt, he recommends practicing poses in the following order: standing, sitting, kneeling, supine, prone, inverted, and relaxing. My teacher usually has us practice inverted poses after standing poses or at the end of class, just before the final relaxing pose. Every yoga teacher has her own interpretations of and variations on the poses, so you might find that your teacher follows a different pose sequence, focuses on just a few types of poses each class, or practices breathing exercises after poses. The important thing to remember is to do what feels right for you.

The Sun Salute series (pages 160–65) can be a complete workout in itself, so you might want to practice it at a separate time, after warming up.

While you practice, keep in mind that yoga's benefits are gained through slow, deliberate movements and breathing, as well as resting. Take a minute to rest in between poses to allow your body to balance itself. If you're like most people, used to hurrying to your next appointment, jumping around in aerobics classes, and running laps around a track, slowing down will be a challenge.

The best way to stay disciplined about practicing is to set aside ten to thirty minutes each day or night for yoga. Some people prefer practicing in the early evening or before sunrise. I like to practice yoga between nine and ten A.M. because it helps me wake up, or at the end of the day to counteract all the hours I've spent sitting in front of my computer. Find a time and place that works for you.

I have listed the poses by category for organizational purposes, but to create a well-rounded routine, you will not necessarily practice them in the order in which they are listed. After completing your breathing and warm-up exercises, you can select a 5–10-, 10–15-, 15–20-, 20–30-, or 30–40-minute workout on pages 168–70. You can also make up your own routines using the criteria I mentioned at the top of the page.

In the back of the book (pages 171–82), I have also listed poses that will help prepare you for different physical activities and sports, as well as poses to practice for different health conditions and poses that benefit specific areas of the body.

Benefits of Poses

The chart below explains the general benefits of different types of yoga poses.

What Different Actions Do for the Body

Abdominal

- Poses that strengthen the abdominal and lower back muscles help keep the pelvis in its neutral position, improving posture. Poses that massage the abdomen improve digestion and the absorption of nutrients in the digestive system.

Backward Bends and Forward Bends

- Backward bends are energizing poses that increase flexibility in the lower spine, open up the front of the body, and increase circulation and respiration.

- Forward bends are relaxing poses that help tone and massage the internal organs, strengthen and stretch the spine, and calm the mind.

Inverted

- Inverted poses counteract our normal upright position and the effects of gravity. These poses increase blood flow to the brain, activating the pituitary and pineal glands, which stimulate the functioning of the endocrine system. Inverted poses also relieve swelling in the legs.

Lying Down (Supine and Prone)

- Supine and prone poses relax the mind and body, promoting improved breath control. Many prone poses involve backward bends, which strengthen and improve flexibility in the spine. Supine poses stretch and strengthen the back and hips.

Relaxing

- Relaxing poses allow the body to come into balance and rest after movement.

Sitting and Kneeling

- Sitting and kneeling poses are ideal for meditation because they relax the mind and calm the nervous system, improving breath control. Sitting and kneeling poses also strengthen the lower back and sacrum area, limber the legs and hips, and promote balance and stability.

Standing

- Standing poses strengthen legs, ankles, feet, hips, and abdominal muscles; develop balance, coordination, and endurance; and improve alignment, circulation, and breathing.

Twists

- Spinal twists help regulate the peristaltic movement of the intestines and bowel, improve digestion, increase spinal flexibility, and stimulate internal organs.

YOGASPEAK

One of yoga's primary benefits is to achieve and maintain correct alignment, so I have described below what alignment looks like in different parts of the body, and during different types of poses. Take time to read this section carefully, trying to visualize what it looks and feels like for your body to be in alignment. Also, familiarizing yourself with the yoga terms that I have defined will make the pose instructions easier to follow.

When the instructions say	It means
Bend at the hips	In forward bends, the goal is to bend from the hips, not from the middle of the back. You want to maintain your spinal alignment during the pose, so focus your energy on relaxing the hip joints so that your body bends forward without the back curving. (See illustration.)

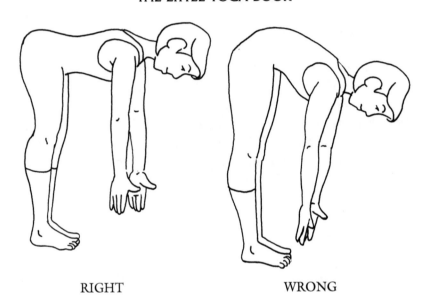

RIGHT   WRONG

Enter deeper into pose   This means increase the level of
intensity (i.e., stretch more deep-
ly), or push yourself to hold the
pose a bit longer than you think
you can. Using your breath to
help relax your body and focus

your mind will help you maintain the pose.

Head Alignment

Maintaining correct spinal alignment involves the top of the spine, as well as the tailbone area (and in between). If you put your hand on the back of your neck and tilt your head backward and forward, you can feel how the back of your neck arches and straightens. The goal is to have your upper spine come straight out of your shoulder area and into the base of your head, with your head resting at the top, eyes looking straight ahead. If you visualize someone pulling up on a string that runs through your spine and out the top of your head, you can experience what proper head alignment feels like. Your

43

chin won't jut out or be perfectly parallel to the floor, but slightly tucked. As you practice head alignment, you can feel the back of your neck straighten and your head tilt into its optimal position.

Hips aligned

Maintaining pelvic alignment means that when you move, you want both of your hips to be in line with each other on horizontal and vertical planes. For example, when you do the Tree pose (page 83), you will be bending one leg while balancing on the other. The trick to maintaining that balance is to have your body in optimal alignment. You want both hips facing forward, aligned with your torso and shoulders, and the same distance from the floor. (That means that one hip isn't cocked higher than the other.) The same is true in the Cat pose Variation (page 126). As you extend your arm and leg, trying to maintain balance, make sure that you are not twisting your pelvis around to hold up your leg. Both hips should be facing the floor, and the same distance from the floor. My friend reminds herself to maintain hip alignment by thinking of her hips as car headlights (i.e., the beams never cross each other, but always remain parallel.)

Hold pose for three to six breaths

Remain in the pose while focusing on your breathing. A breath consists of one inhalation and one exhalation.

In a standing position

Stand straight and tall, lifting the spine out of the pelvis as if there were a string coming out the top of your head and being pulled into the sky. Point your tailbone downward. Engage your abdominal muscles, which helps tip the pelvis into its correct alignment or "neutral position." Relax your shoulders, pulling them down, away from your ears, and press your shoulder blades flat against your back. Relax the arms, allowing them to hang at your sides. Relax the buttock muscles. Engage the thighs, pulling up on the kneecaps. Knees should not be locked. Your toes should be spread apart and your feet firmly planted on the floor (See Mountain pose on page 75.) (See illustration.)

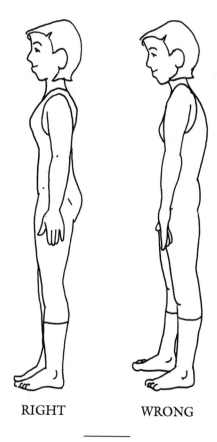

RIGHT   WRONG

In a sitting position

Maintain the same posture as in a standing position, but sit cross-legged on the floor or with legs extended in front of you. (See illustration.)

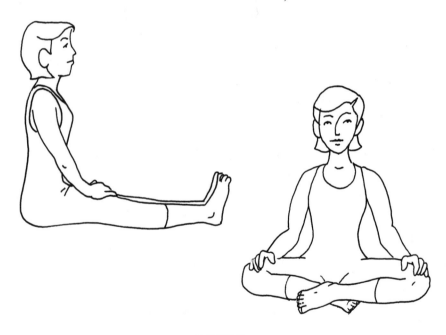

Neutral position

Neutral position refers to any pose or movement that places a body part, particularly the pelvis or spine, in optimal alignment. It is "neutral" because holding the body in this position requires less energy and allows the most free and efficient movement.

Keep legs straight

Straight legs support the body's weight through strength and balance. A common mistake is to lock your knees when standing. By engaging your thigh muscles and gently pulling up on your kneecaps, you will be able to straighten your legs (without locking your knees) and to feel how your leg muscles support your weight. The next step is to spread your toes apart and anchor them to the ground, shifting your weight over the center of your feet.

Keep shoulders down

In poses where you reach your arms over your head, like the Half Moon pose (page 78), it is important to maintain proper alignment in your upper back. A common mistake is scrunching up your shoulders when you raise arms. As in other poses, optimal posture will allow your body to do the stretch the most efficient way. Keeping your shoulders pulled down away from your ears and your shoulder blades pressed flat against your back will ultimately free your arms to stretch higher above your head. (See illustration.)

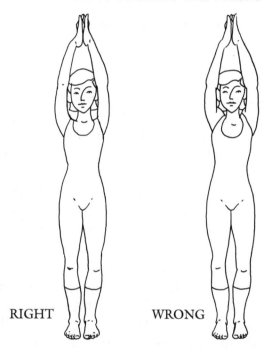

RIGHT   WRONG

Lift spine out of pelvis   Elongate your spine in your lower back and stretch the sides of your torso, lifting the body upward.

DEFINITION OF TERMS

Alignment

- What makes yoga so challenging is maintaining alignment throughout the body while doing poses. In addition to spinal alignment, the body must be aligned in space. In other words, body parts should be aligned with other body parts, as well as in the same plane. For example, during the Warrior pose (page 95), the knee and foot of the bent leg should be in alignment, forming a straight line at a 90° angle with the floor. And in the Half Moon pose (page 78), the arms should be raised above the head, palms together and pointing upward. Arms, ears, torso, and legs should all be in a straight line. Visualize that you are doing the pose between two invisible walls that are only a foot apart to keep yourself from sticking your head forward or your butt backward.

Belly

- The area below your navel.

Counterpose

- A pose that provides a stretch in the opposite direction of the pose preceding it. Counterposes for the back are important in developing strength and flexibility in balanced proportions. For example, if you practice a pose like the Cobra that arches your back, follow it with a pose like the Child's or the Head to Knee that rounds the back.

Engaging

- The gentle contracting of muscles (such as leg and abdominal) during a pose. This action provides support, promotes posture, and keeps body parts actively involved in a pose.

Limber

- To gently stretch and loosen.

Massage

- Many poses "massage" different internal organs. Massage means that the pose's breathing and movements stimulate the organs, increasing blood flow to the area and improving functioning.

Neutral spine

- See "In a standing position."

Open

- An "opening" of the body occurs when a muscle or area is expanded, stretched, or released.

Poses

- The positions, or postures, involved in yoga exercise. Also called asanas.

Prone

- Lying on your stomach.

Release

- To let go of tightness or tension. When bending or stretching, it helps to visualize the tight area releasing or letting go. Focusing your breath on the tight area helps. Releasing also means letting go of negative thoughts like, "I can't do this pose."

Supine

- Lying on your back.

6/The Poses

A Lifetime of Yoga

There are hundreds (some say thousands) of yoga poses, so there's plenty to keep you busy for a lifetime of practice. Your teacher can help you select a combination of poses for your home practice, and there is a list of sample workouts in the back of this book (pages 168–70).

All of the breathing exercises, warm-ups, and poses have been reviewed for accuracy and safety by a certified yoga teacher with over twenty-five years of teaching experience.

Some of the poses here may be slightly different from what you've seen in other books or learned in class. You'll notice after taking a few classes that every teacher (and student) adds her own style and variations to each pose.

I've tried to describe the poses in their simplest forms to allow you room to make your own adaptations. I have not included headstands because they can be dangerous for beginning and intermediate level students and should be practiced only by advanced students under the guidance and supervision of an experienced teacher. Also, you will notice that in order to keep the exercises safe and simple, I don't recommend in my instructions arching the back or neck in backward bending poses.

I hope that this book has helped dispel some myths about yoga and helped you get started in your own yoga practice. Take your time, enjoy yourself, and keeping bending.

How to Follow the Instructions

After you have read the first part of the book and are ready to begin exercising, studying the instructions for each pose carefully and reviewing the terms in Yogaspeak will help you prepare mentally for practice. All of the poses in this section follow the same easy-to-use format:

Name of pose:

Where available I have listed the Sanskrit names for the poses after the common English names. Because everyone who teaches and studies yoga makes his or her own practice unique, adapting styles or creating variations, it is common to see the same pose named and practiced differently in different sources.

Benefits:

This section briefly mentions the primary physical and mental benefits that each pose imparts.

Instructions:

Read each step carefully before practicing a pose, using the illustrations as guidelines. The illustrations are meant to show the essence of the pose, so for exact details on placement and breathing, follow the written instructions. It you have any problems or can't remember how to do a pose, ask your teacher to demonstrate it for you. When the instructions mention breathing, it means to breathe normally, inhaling and exhaling freely, unless otherwise noted. As you become more experienced, your teacher can show you how to enter deeper into a pose by breathing more slowly and deeply.

Tips:

This section tells you additional information about the pose or variations on the pose. As a general guideline, I have also indicated here where in your body you are likely to feel the stretch as you do the pose. Because everyone's body experiences yoga differently, you might feel stretches, tightness, or other sensations as you exercise that I haven't listed.

Rating:

All of the poses are rated I (for simpler poses) or II (for more challenging poses). These ratings are only guidelines. Everyone's body is different. Depending on your experience, health, body type, and fitness level, you might be able to do more or less than the instructions describe. For example, a beginner might be able to do a level II pose with ease, and an intermediate level person might find certain level I poses challenging. Listen to your body to determine which poses you feel comfortable practicing. A I & II rating means that the pose is appropriate for both levels. Remember, yoga is not a competition. Even the most advanced yoga student still benefits from practicing level I poses, and a well-rounded practice will contain level I and level II poses.

Cautions:

This section notes existing health conditions that might be aggravated by the pose. If you are on medication or have any of the following health conditions, ask your doctor and teacher to help you determine which poses are safe for you to do: high blood pressure, back or neck pain, heart problems, pregnancy, vertigo. The more information your teacher has about your health, the better she can help you find a routine that's most beneficial to your needs. The best way to prevent injury is to listen to your body and do only what feels right to you.

POSES (ASANAS)

Warm-ups

Shoulder Roll
Neck Stretch
Foot Stretch
Arm Reach
Arm Stretch

Standing Poses

Mountain
Half Moon
Dancer
Tree
Triangle
Twisting Triangle
Standing Knee Squeeze
Standing Forward Bend

Warrior
Eagle

Seated Poses

Seated Arm Stretch
Butterfly
Seated Forward Bend
Spinal Twist
Side Bend Over Legs
Head to Knee

Kneeling Poses

Thunderbolt
Pigeon
Kneeling Chest Expander

Cowhead
Cat
Downward Facing Dog

Lying Down Poses
(Supine, Prone)

Leg Lifts
Knees to Chest
Lying Down Twists
Bridge
Fish
Locust and Half Locust
Cobra

Inverted Poses

Plough
Simple Inverted

Relaxing Poses

Child's pose
Relaxing pose

Series Poses

Sun Salute

WARM-UPS

As I mentioned on page 36, your yoga practice will consist of three steps: breathing exercises, warm-up exercises, and poses. After completing a few breathing exercises, these warm-up exercises will prepare you for the main poses.

Shoulder Roll

Benefits:

Loosens shoulder joints and upper back, improves posture.

Instructions:

1. In a standing pose, inhale, lifting shoulders toward ears.
2. Exhale, pulling shoulders back, then dropping them.
3. Repeat pose five times.

Tips:

- Keep arms and neck loose and relaxed.

- Maintain neutral spine.

- You will feel a stretch in the base of your neck.

Rating: I

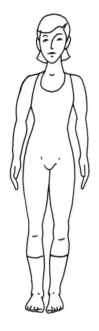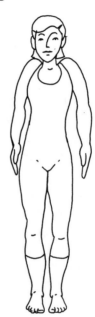

Neck Stretch

Benefits:

Stretches neck muscles, reducing tension in neck.

Instructions:

1. In a standing pose, exhale, gently letting head fall to right side. Hold pose for two to three breaths.
2. Inhale, slowly lifting head back to beginning position.
3. Exhale, gently letting head fall to left side. Hold pose for two to three breaths.
4. Inhale, slowly lifting head back to beginning position.
5. Exhale, gently letting head fall forward. Hold pose for two to three breaths.
6. Inhale, slowly lifting head back to beginning position. Exhale, gently letting head fall backward. Hold pose for two to three breaths.
7. Inhale, slowly returning head to upright position. Repeat pose two to three times.

Tips:

- Keep shoulders relaxed and down from ears, shoulder blades flat against back.

- Keep arms relaxed.

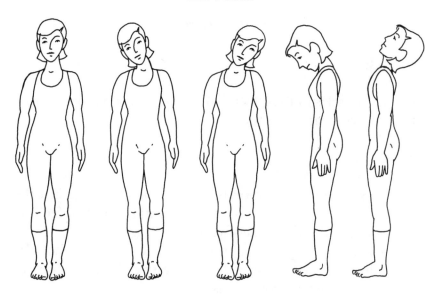

- You will feel a stretch in the sides, front, and back of your neck.

Rating: I

Caution:
- Be careful if you have neck problems.

Foot Stretch

Benefits:

Stretches muscles in toes, feet, ankles, and shins. Warms feet by improving circulation to them.

Instructions:

1. In a kneeling pose, sit on heels with toes flexed against the floor. Hold pose for three to six breaths. You will feel the stretch in the bottoms of your feet.
2. In a kneeling pose, sit on heels with tops of feet flat against the floor. You will feel the stretch at the tops of your feet and up your shins.
3. With left hand, lift left knee off of floor until you feel a stretch in the top of your left foot. Hold pose for three to six breaths.
4. Repeat on opposite side.

Tip:

- Be gentle with yourself. This pose is simple, but it provides a deep stretch.

Rating: I

Caution:

- Be careful if you have knee problems.

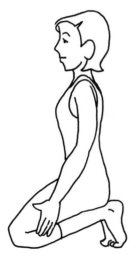
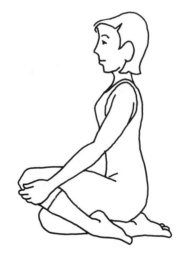

Arm Reach

Benefits:

Loosens shoulder joints and stretches upper back.

Instructions:

1. In a standing pose, inhale and put arms in the air, reaching toward the ceiling.
2. Exhale, allowing shoulders to return to normal position, and dropping arms to sides.
3. Repeat pose five times.

Tips:

- Maintain correct head alignment, eyes looking straight ahead.

- You will feel a stretch in your shoulder blades.

Rating: I

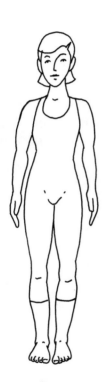

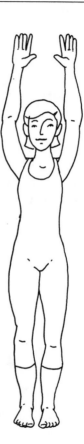

Arm Stretch

Benefits:

Stretches and strengthens arms and wrists.

Instructions:

1. Starting in a kneeling pose, lean forward and put hands on floor in front of you, with hands aligned underneath shoulders and fingers spread apart and pointing forward.

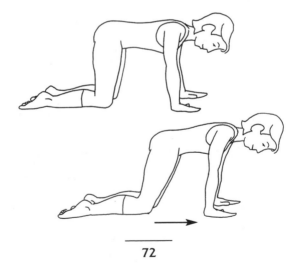

2. Slowly lean over hands until you feel a stretch in the fronts and backs of wrists. Hold pose for two to three breaths.
3. Return to beginning position. Repeat pose three times.
4. Switch direction of hands so that insides of wrists are facing forward and fingertips are pointing toward knees.

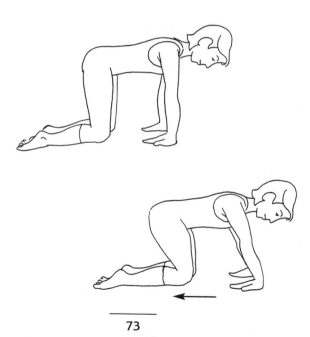

5. Slowly lean backward, pulling hips toward feet as if to sit on heels, keeping hands on floor, until you feel a stretch in your arms and wrists. Hold pose two to three breaths. Repeat pose three times.
6. Counterpose this stretch by shaking hands to loosen wrists.

Tips:
- This is a good exercise for computer users.

- You will feel a stretch in your wrists, arms, and tops of your hands.

Rating: I

STANDING POSES

Mountain (Tadasana)

The Mountain pose, one of the most basic yoga exercises, forms the foundation for many other poses because it sets the standard for spinal alignment. Once you understand what it feels like to achieve correct alignment throughout your body, you can apply this knowledge to other poses and to activities in your daily life.

Benefits:

Strengthens legs and abdominal muscles, improves balance and coordination.

Instructions:

1. Stand with legs together, ankles and feet touching each other.
2. Engage thigh muscles, gently pulling up on kneecaps. Do not lock knees.
3. Gently engage abdominal muscles, pointing the tailbone downward. (Notice how the pelvis tips slightly backward into neutral position.) Relax buttock muscles.
4. Allow arms and shoulders to hang at sides, slightly lifting the chest and tucking shoulder blades flat against back.
5. Maintain correct head alignment, eyes looking straight ahead.
6. Hold pose for three to six breaths.

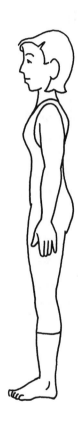

Tips:
- Keep pelvis in neutral position.

- Spread toes to help with balance and support.

- Keep neck, shoulders, and arms relaxed.

- Visualize your spine as straight and tall, as if someone were pulling up on a string attached to the top of your head.

- You will feel this pose in your abdominal muscles, feet, legs, lower back, and chest.

Rating: I

Cautions:
- Standing poses are strenuous and sometimes cause dizziness. You can counteract this by breathing continuously. If this doesn't relieve your dizziness, squat, sit down, or lie on the floor in Relaxing pose (page 158) and rest until you feel better.

Half Moon (Ardha-chandrasana)

Benefits:

Stretches and lengthens sides of torso, increases spinal flexibility, loosens legs and hips, massages liver and spleen, and stimulates digestion.

Instructions:

1. From a standing pose, inhale, raising arms over head, palms together.
2. Exhale, slowly leaning and stretching to left side, pointing tips of fingers up and to the left.
3. Hold pose for three to six breaths.
4. Inhale, returning to standing pose. Repeat on opposite side.
5. Return to standing pose. Repeat pose two to three times.

Tips:

- Keep hips aligned.

- Keep arms even with ears.

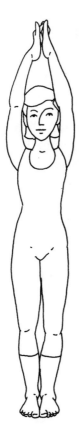

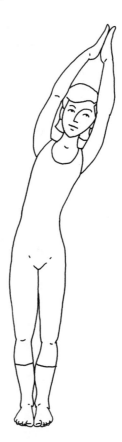

- Maintain correct head alignment, eyes looking straight ahead.

- Keep shoulders down, away from ears and relaxed.

- You will feel a stretch through the sides of your torso, and in your feet, legs, abdominal muscles, and back.

Rating: I

Cautions:
- May cause dizziness.

- Be careful if you have back problems.

Dancer (Natarajasana)

Benefits:

Strengthens muscles in the legs, feet, and lower back, improves balance and concentration, stretches and opens the hips and pelvis, and strengthens the psoas muscles (the muscles that connect the torso to the lower body).

Instructions:

1. In a standing pose, bend left knee, raising left foot up to buttocks.
2. Hold left ankle (or left foot) with left hand. Raise right hand in the air, balancing on your right foot.
3. Hold pose for three to six breaths. Repeat on opposite side.
4. Return to standing pose. Repeat pose two to three times.

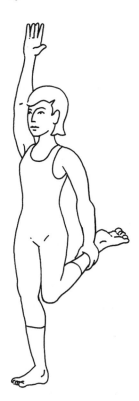

Tips:

- Fix your eyes on a point in front of you to aid in balance.

- Stand close to the wall if unsteady.

- Keep toes of standing leg pointed forward, foot flat on the floor.

- Relax stomach muscles and breathe normally.

- You will feel a stretch in the thigh of your lifted leg.

- Using a full, steady Ujjayi breath will help you stay focused and balanced.

Rating: II

Caution:

- Be careful if you have back or foot problems.

Tree (Vrksasana)

Benefits:

Strengthens legs and ankles, opens hips, and improves balance, coordination, and concentration.

Instructions:

1. Start in standing pose.
2. Bend left knee, take left foot with hands, and rest left side of left foot on the top of the right leg thigh. (If this is too difficult, place sole of left foot against inside upper thigh of right leg.)
3. Raise arms in air above head, palms together.

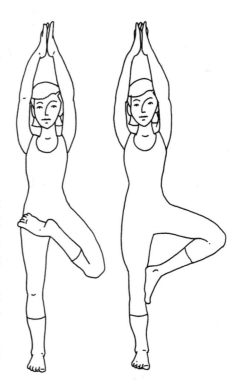

4. Hold pose for three to six breaths.
5. Repeat on opposite side. Return to standing pose. Repeat pose two to three times.

Tips:

• Keep arms straight.

• If you have difficulty with step 2, hold foot as close to position as you can with opposite hand.

• Fix your eyes on a point in front of you to aid in balance.

• Stand close to the wall if unsteady.

• Relax stomach muscles.

• You will feel a stretch in your hip, thigh, knee of bent leg, and in ankles.

Rating: I & II

Cautions:
- May cause dizziness.

- Be careful if you have knee or ankle problems.

Triangle (Trikonasana)

Benefits:

Firms thigh, calf, and hamstring muscles of the legs, strengthens hip and ankle muscles, and improves balance. Stretches arms, back, shoulders, and sides of torso. Stimulates abdominal organs and increases spinal flexibility.

Instructions:

VARIATION A:

1. From a standing position with arms hanging at sides, raise arms parallel to floor and even with shoulders, and spread feet apart about four feet.
2. Turn left foot out, so it points in the same direction as left hand, and heel of left foot is perpendicular to arch of right foot. Turn right foot 30° to the left.
3. Square the hips so that they are facing forward. Inhale.
4. Exhale, slowly bending over to the left side until the fingertips of your left hand are touching the floor on the inside of your left foot.
5. Right arm will be vertical, fingers pointing to the ceiling.
6. Turn head so that eyes are focused on raised hand. Hold pose for three to six breaths.
7. To come out of pose, inhale while you place right hand on right hip, bend left knee and place left hand on left knee. Slowly push up left arm, straighten leg, and return to standing pose.
8. Repeat on opposite side. Repeat pose two to three times.

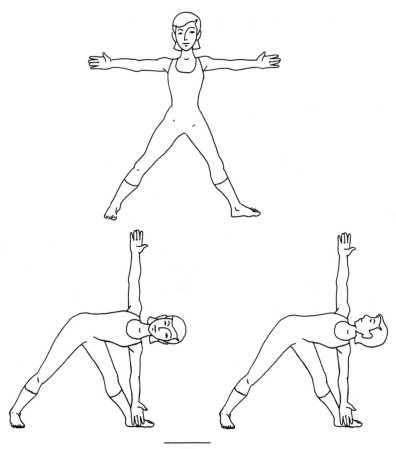

Twisting Triangle (Parivrtta Trikonasana)

VARIATION B:

1. From a standing position with arms hanging at sides, raise arms parallel to floor and even with shoulders, and spread feet apart about four feet.
2. Turn left foot out, so it points in the same direction as left hand, and heel of left foot is perpendicular to arch of right foot. Turn right foot 30° to the left.
3. With inhaling breath, lift the spine out of the pelvis and shift weight over left leg.
4. From that position, exhale and twist at the hips and rotate, bringing the right hand to the left foot or ankle. Left arm will be pointing toward the ceiling. Turn head so that eyes are focused on raised hand. Hold pose for three to six breaths.
5. Come out of pose slowly by resting hands on floor in front of you, turning left foot forward. Inhale as you bend knees and with hands supporting lower back, stand up. Repeat on opposite side. Repeat pose two to three times.

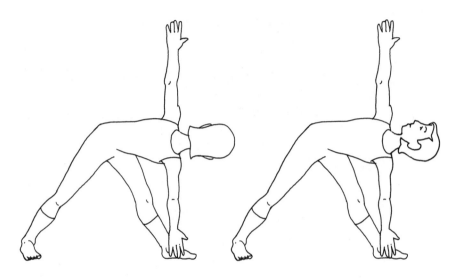

Tips:
- Maintain correct hip alignment.

- Go slowly, and remember to keep breathing.

- If you can, keep legs straight, and if you can't touch the floor in step 4, reach as far as you can.

- Using a slow, steady inhaling breath while coming out of pose will minimize dizziness.

- If you feel unsteady, use a wall for support.

- You will feel a stretch in the sides of your torso, lower back, and knees.

Rating: II

Caution:
- Be careful if you have back problems.

Standing Knee Squeeze (Pavanmuktasana)

Benefits:

Strengthens lower back, hips, spine, and legs, and improves balance, posture, and concentration.

Instructions:

1. From a standing pose, raise right knee and interlock fingers around leg, pulling it to body in a gentle hug.
2. Hold pose for three to six breaths. Release leg with an exhaling breath.
3. Repeat on opposite side. Repeat pose two to three times.

Tips:

- Relax foot and ankle of raised leg.

- Keep shoulders down, spine in neutral position.

- You will feel a stretch in your lower back and shoulders.

Rating: I

Caution:

- Be careful if you have knee or back problems.

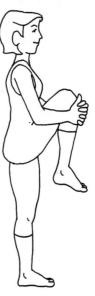

Standing Forward Bend (Padahastasana)

Benefits:

Loosens hamstrings, strengthens legs, massages pelvic organs, calms the nervous system, and increases blood flow to head and face. Stretches and strengthens the spine.

Instructions:

1. In a standing pose, inhale and bend knees several inches.
2. Exhale, bending at the hips and placing stomach on top of thighs and chest near knees. Hold on to ankles or lower legs with hands, tucking elbows behind calves (or behind knees if you have long arms). Allow head to relax and dangle toward the floor.
3. Keep breathing.
4. Slowly, with each exhaling breath, extend the tailbone upward and try to straighten legs, keeping stomach and chest on thighs.
5. Hold pose for three to six breaths.

6. Come out of pose slowly. Touch the floor with hands. With an inhaling breath, bend knees slightly and slide hands up legs from ankles to knees. Rest hands on top of knees, exhale. Inhale, sliding hands up thighs until you reach your hips. Tuck tailbone downward and raise body into upright position. Repeat pose two to three times.

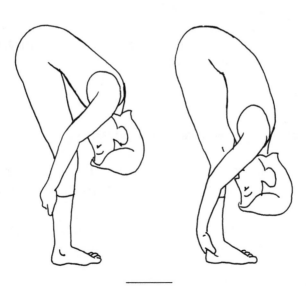

Tips:
- Try to maintain neutral spine, and when you bend, release from the hips.

- The goal is to stretch lower back and hamstrings, so don't worry if you can't straighten your legs.

- Maintaining steady breathing will minimize dizziness.

- You will feel a stretch in your hamstrings and lower back.

Rating: II

Cautions:
- May cause dizziness.

- Do not do this pose if you feel throbbing in your temples when you bend over.

Warrior (Virasana)

Benefits:

Strengthens back, legs, hips, arms and shoulders, stretches groin and leg muscles. Opens chest and improves balance and stamina.

Instructions:

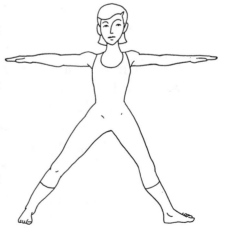

1. Stand with feet approximately three to four feet apart, extending arms parallel to floor, palms down.
2. Turn left foot out, so it points in the same direction as left hand, and heel of left foot is perpendicular to arch of right foot. Square the hips so that they are facing forward. Inhale.

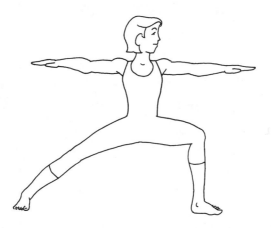

3. Bend left knee, lowering body into a lunge position over left foot. Left knee and foot should be in alignment, forming a 90° angle with floor. You may have to readjust your position, spreading feet wider apart, to achieve this alignment. Keep hips aligned.
4. Turn head to the left, looking past left hand.
5. Hold pose for three to six breaths.
6. Repeat on opposite side. Repeat pose two to three times.

Tips:
- Keep hips and shoulders aligned and facing forward.

- Keep arms and shoulders relaxed.

- You will feel a stretch in your inner thighs, thigh of bent leg, shoulders, and calf of straight leg.

Rating: I

Caution:
- Be careful if you have knee problems.

Eagle (Garudasana)

Benefits:

Stretches shoulders, strengthens legs and ankles, improves balance, concentration, and coordination.

Instructions:

1. In a standing pose, cross right leg over left leg, tucking right foot behind calf of left leg.
2. Raise arms parallel to floor and even with shoulders.
3. Hug yourself, placing right arm above left arm, and grasping shoulder blades.
4. Keeping right elbow resting against left elbow, lift right forearm into a vertical position.
5. Wind left arm around right arm until you are grasping right palm with left fingers. Fingers will be pointing toward the ceiling. As you inhale, raise arms up and look up at fingers. Hold pose three to six breaths.
6. Exhale and allow arms to drop down to your sides. Uncross legs. Repeat on opposite side. Repeat pose two to three times.

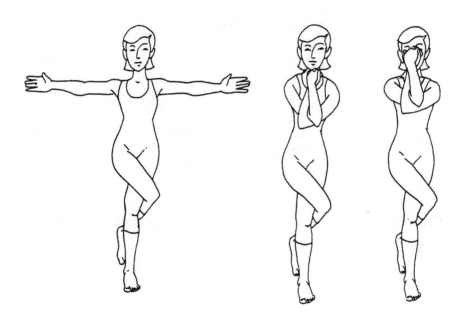

Tips:
- To modify pose, start in kneeling position, sitting on heels, and follow steps two through six.

- Don't arch lower back.

- Maintain neutral spine by engaging abdominal muscles and pointing tailbone downward.

- You will feel a stretch in your upper back, hips, and ankles.

Rating: II

Caution:
- Be careful if you have back problems.

SEATED POSES

Seated Arm Stretch (Parvatasana)

Benefits:

Stretches shoulders, arms, and upper back.

Instructions:

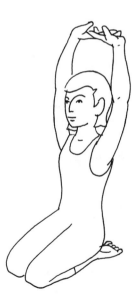

1. In a kneeling position, or in a seated position with legs crossed and arms resting on legs, interlock fingers in front of body.
2. Inhale, raising arms over your head, keeping your shoulders down. Turn interlocked palms upward, pointing and reaching them toward ceiling.
3. Exhale, relaxing stretch by bending arms, then releasing fingers and slowly lowering arms to sides. Repeat pose two to three times.

Tips:
- Good for computer users.

- Arms should be aligned with ears.

- You will feel a stretch in your wrists and between your shoulder blades.

Rating: I

Butterfly (Upavistha Konasana)

Benefits:

Opens and stretches the groin area, improving blood and lymph circulation in the legs.

Instructions:

1. In a seated position with bent knees and soles of feet touching, interlock fingers and hold feet across tops of toes. Inhale.
2. Exhale, lifting knees up.
3. Inhale, lowering knees to floor.
4. Repeat five times.

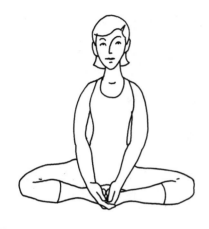 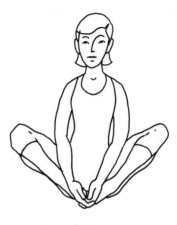

Tips:

• Maintain neutral spine.

• Keep sides of feet against floor.

• If you cannot lower knees to floor, lower them as far as you can.

• You will feel a stretch in your groin, inner thighs, and hips.

Rating: I & II

Seated Forward Bend (Paschimottanasana)

Benefits:

Lengthens spine, opens back, and massages internal organs.

Instructions:

1. In a seated position with legs together and extended, inhale, reaching arms over head. Toes should be pointed upward.
2. Exhale, bending at the hips and leaning out over legs. Look at ankles or past tops of toes.
3. Hold legs or ankles, keeping spine straight, for three to six breaths. If you can, rest your head on your knees.
4. With each exhaling breath, try to release hips further, bending deeper into the stretch.
5. Inhale as you raise arms over head and return to an upright position. Exhale, dropping arms to sides. Repeat pose two to three times.

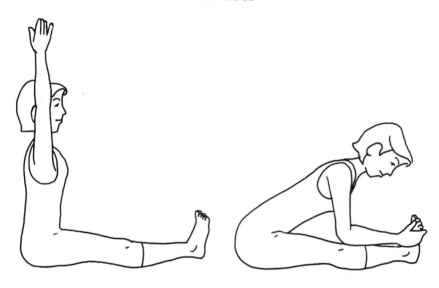

Tips:

- Keep shoulders down, away from ears.

- Keep legs engaged.

- Bend at hips, not at middle back. It's more important to maintain correct posture than to get your chest close to your legs.

- If you can't hold on to your ankles, hold your legs as close to your ankles as you can.

- You will feel a stretch in your lower back and hamstrings.

Rating: I & II

Cautions: • May cause dizziness.

- Be careful if you have back problems.

Spinal Twist (Ardha Matsendrasana)

Benefits:

Realigns the vertebrae, adding strength and flexibility to the spine, and massages internal organs, improving liver and kidney functions and digestion. Twists also stretch and strengthen arms, shoulders, and neck muscles.

Instructions:

1. From a sitting position, extend left leg and bend right leg over left leg so that right foot rests against left hip.*
2. Holding on to bent leg and hugging it to body with left arm, inhale and lift the spine out of the pelvis. Put right hand on the floor behind buttocks for support, fingers

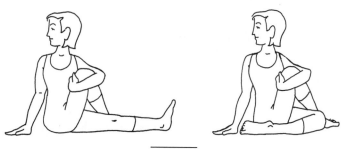

pointing backward. (You will probably have to raise your fingers to maintain contact with the floor.)

3. As you exhale, turn your body to the right, keeping spine straight and tall, and turn your head over your right shoulder until you are looking behind yourself. Hold pose for three to six breaths.

4. Repeat for opposite side. Repeat pose two to three times.

Tips:
- Sit on small cushion to help take stress off of back and knees.

- If you can't do step 1, place foot close to thigh or knees.

- Keep spine straight and tall. Keep extended leg engaged.

- You will feel a stretch in your back, hips, and neck.

Rating: II

*For a more difficult pose, begin pose by bending the left leg back until foot touches right hip. Then, bend right leg over left thigh until right foot rests against left hip. (See second figure.)

Caution: • Be careful if you have neck or shoulder problems.

Side Bend Over Legs
(Parsva Upavistha Konasana)

Benefits:

Stretches inner thighs, sides of torso, hips, and pelvic muscles.

Instructions:

1. Sit with legs extended and open wide (forming a "V"), feet flexed and toes pointing upward.
2. Reach arms upward, inhaling.
3. Exhale, turning body to right.
4. Bend at hips, extending body over right leg. Rest arms on floor or hold on to foot if you can reach that far. Look straight ahead at foot.

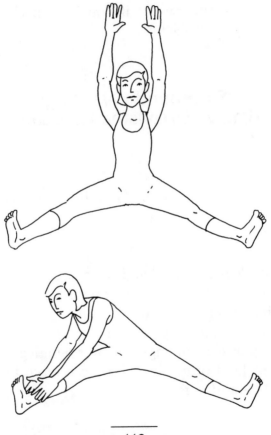

5. Hold pose for three to six breaths.
6. Inhale, slowly raising body from the hips and rolling spine back into sitting position, using arms as support.
7. Repeat on opposite side. Repeat pose two to three times.

Tips:
- You can sit on a small cushion to make pose easier.

- Keep shoulders relaxed and legs engaged.

- You will feel a stretch in your hamstrings, inner thighs, and lower back.

Rating: II

Caution:
- Be careful if you have neck or back problems.

Head to Knee (Janu Sirsasana)

Benefits:

Stimulates the kidneys, liver, and pancreas, stretches and strengthens the leg muscles, stimulates blood circulation to the spine, and calms the nervous system.

Instructions:

1. Sit with right leg extended in front of body. Bend left leg and place foot against inside of right thigh.
2. Inhale, interlocking fingers of both hands with palms facing toward right foot.
3. Exhale, extending hands along right leg toward your right foot in a scooping motion as you bend from hips over your right leg.
4. When hands reach foot, inhale, raising arms in the air over head with hands still interlocked and returning to an upright, seated position (interlocked hands will be above head, palms up). Lift spine out of pelvis.

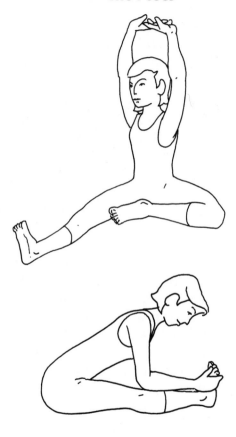

5. Exhale, bending at the hips and extending body out over right leg. Grasp ankle. Hold pose for three to six breaths.

6. Inhale, pulling hands along right leg and slowly raise the torso from the hips, one vertebra at a time, until in a sitting position again.

7. Repeat with left leg extended and right leg bent with foot resting against left leg. Repeat pose two to three times.

Tips:

- Keep extended leg engaged.

- Maintain neutral spine by engaging abdominal muscles and pointing tailbone downward.

- It's better to maintain correct posture and not be able to bend all the way down or reach your ankle than to reach your ankle and let your back hunch over.

- You will feel a stretch in your lower back, hamstrings, and upper body.

Rating: II

KNEELING POSES

Thunderbolt (Vajrasana)

Benefits:

Calms the mind and relaxes the body in preparation for meditation, breathing exercises, or other kneeling poses.

Instructions:

1. Kneel on floor with buttocks between feet, thighs together, keeping the spine straight. If you can't sit between your feet, sit on a small cushion or on your heels.
2. Place hands on knees, palms down.
3. Hold pose for five breaths.

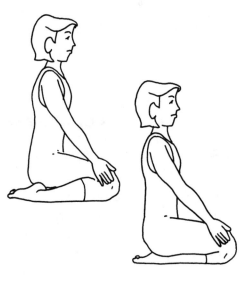

Tips:
- Maintain neutral spine by engaging abdominal muscles and pointing tailbone downward.

- You will feel a stretch in your knees, thighs, ankles, and hips.

Rating: I

Caution:
- Be careful if you have knee problems.

Pigeon (Rajakapotasana)

Benefits:

Stretches and strengthens spine, hips, groin, and opens chest. The backward and forward bending actions in this pose massage adrenal glands and kidneys.

Instructions:

1. Sit in a kneeling pose with heels underneath buttocks and hands on the floor next to knees. Inhale.
2. Exhale, extending right leg behind body and laying chest across left thigh. Place forehead on floor.
3. Inhale, lifting upper body one vertebra at a time from the base of the spine. Use arms for support. You will end up sitting on your left foot.
4. Look straight ahead, maintaining correct head alignment. If you have short arms, you may need to extend your fingers so that you can still maintain contact with floor.
5. Hold pose for three to six breaths. Repeat on opposite side. Repeat pose two to three times.

Tips:
- Use arms and hands for support, not to lift upper body.

- Keep hips aligned.

- You will feel a stretch in front of hips and in lower back.

Rating: II

Caution:
- Be careful if you have lower back problems.

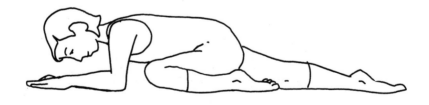

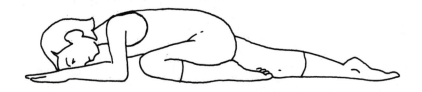

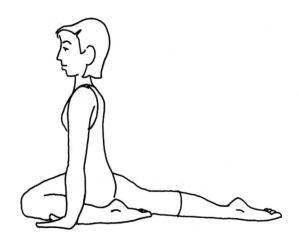

Kneeling Chest Expander (Yogasana)

Benefits:

Stretches and loosens shoulders and spine, and increases circulation to spine and head.

Instructions:

1. From a kneeling pose, sit back on heels with tops of feet flat against floor.
2. Interlock fingers behind back, palms facing your back.
3. Inhale, lifting clasped hands up as high as you can.
4. Hold pose for three to six breaths.
5. Exhale, bend forward over thighs, resting forehead on the floor.
6. Lift clasped hands up as high as you can, this time perpendicular to the floor.
7. Hold pose for three to six breaths. Repeat pose two to three times.

Tips:

- Keep shoulders down and away from ears.

- Maintain neutral spine.

- You will feel a stretch between shoulder blades.

Rating: I

Caution:

- May cause dizziness.

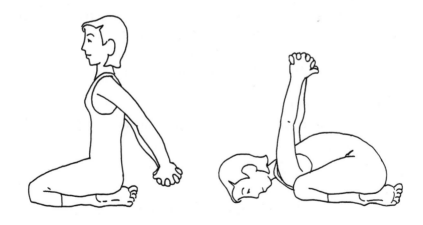

Cowhead (Gomukhasana)

Benefits:

Improves posture by loosening up the shoulder joints and strengthening the muscles in the upper back and arms.

Instructions:

1. From a kneeling position, sit back on heels and let arms hang at sides.
2. Place the back of your right hand on your back, between your shoulder blades, palm facing out.
3. Raise left arm into vertical position, bend at elbow, and try to grasp right hand with left hand so that fingers are hooked underneath each other.
4. Hold pose for three to six breaths.
5. Repeat with opposite side. Repeat pose two to three times.

Tips:
- Don't arch back.

- Maintain neutral spine.

- If you can't grasp your hands, hold a small towel between them to do the stretch.

- Good for computer users.

- You will feel a stretch between your shoulder blades and in your shoulders and arms.

Rating: I & II

Caution:

- Be careful if you have neck or back problems.

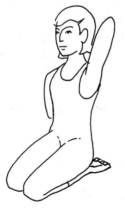 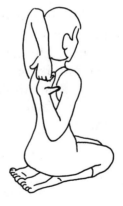

Cat (Marjariasana)

Benefits:

Massages the muscles of the back, improving spinal flexibility and relieving lower back tension, calms the nervous system, and improves circulation. The Cat pose also flattens the stomach, massages the kidneys, and helps remove fat from around the liver. The variation strengthens the hip joints, shoulders, upper back, and improves balance.

Instructions:

1. Starting in a kneeling position, lean forward and place hands on floor underneath shoulders, fingers spread apart and facing forward.
2. With the inhaling breath, slowly extend the tailbone upward, arching spine, dropping stomach toward the floor, and looking up.
3. As you exhale, reverse the pose by arching back the opposite way. Tuck chin into chest and round the spine, tuck-

ing the tailbone downward, as if a string were tied around your waist pulling you up.

4. Repeat pose two to three times.

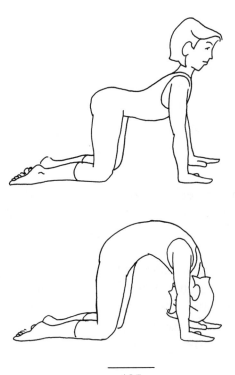

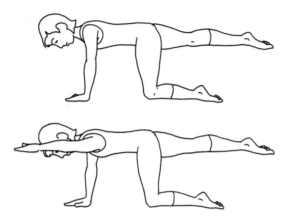

CAT VARIATION:

1. Starting in a kneeling position, lean forward and place hands on floor underneath shoulders, looking straight ahead (or down at floor if that's more comfortable for your neck).
2. Extend right leg parallel to floor, keeping hips aligned.
3. Extend and stretch left arm forward, parallel to floor.
4. Hold pose for three to six breaths. Return arm and leg to kneeling position. Repeat with left leg and right arm. Repeat pose two to three times.

Tips:
- Keep shoulders down and pulled back from ears.

- In Cat variation, keep spine straight and long, with arm and leg in one line parallel to floor. Stretch fingertips forward and toes backward during pose. Keep both hips aligned with the floor (i.e., an equal distance from the floor).

- Fix your eyes on a point in front of you to aid in balance.

- Breathe slowly and deeply, coordinating breath with movement.

- You will feel a stretch in your back, and in the variation, in your shoulders, arms, legs, wrists, hips, and lower back.

Rating: I

Caution:
- Be careful if you have back or neck problems.

Downward Facing Dog
(Adho Mukha Svanasana)

Benefits:

Stretches back, legs, and backs of ankles, opens chest, massages abdominal muscles, and increases circulation to head and face.

Instructions:

1. In a kneeling position, place hands on floor in front of body and directly beneath shoulders.
2. Turn toes under, flexing them against floor. Inhale.
3. Exhale, raising hips into the air, forming an inverted "V".
4. Lift and point tailbone upward while pressing chest toward floor. Drop head between arms toward the floor.
5. If you can, lower heels to floor. Hold pose for three to six breaths.
6. Release pose by coming down on all fours. Repeat pose two to three times.

Tips:
- Keep sinking the upper back (dropping chest toward floor) so that you have a straight back.

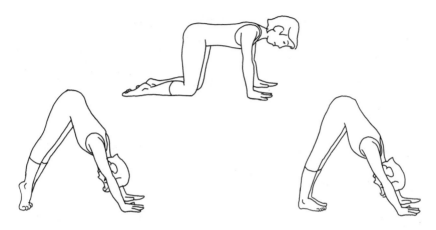

- Keep arms and legs straight, and legs and ankles together.

- If it is too difficult to keep your heels on the floor, keep toes on floor.
- You will feel a stretch at the backs of your legs and in your back, arms, wrists, and shoulders.

Rating: II
Caution:

- May cause dizziness.

LYING DOWN POSES
(SUPINE AND PRONE)

Leg Lifts (Urdhva Prasarita Padasana)

Benefits:

Strengthens abdominal, leg, and back muscles.

Instructions:

1. Lie on your back on the floor with hands at sides, palms down, feet flexed with toes pointing upward.
2. Inhale, extending right heel and lifting right leg off the floor to a 90° angle.
3. Hold pose for three to six breaths.
4. Exhale, slowly lowering right leg to floor.
5. Repeat on opposite side, then repeat at 60° angle and 30° angle for each leg. Repeat pose two to three times.

Tips: • (To modify pose, lie on your back with your knees bent and feet flat on the floor, hands

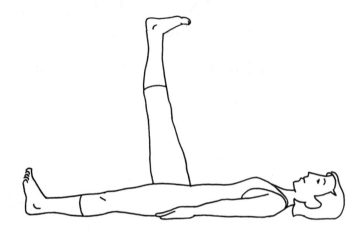

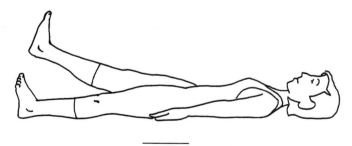

at sides. Extend right leg, with toes of right foot flexed and pointing upward. Then follow the instructions from step 2.)

• Keep lower abdominal muscles engaged.

• When legs are extended, keep them straight, with thigh muscles engaged.

• Lower back will maintain its natural curve, so it will not touch floor.

• You will feel a stretch in your abdominal muscles and thighs.

Rating: II

Caution: • Be careful if you have back problems.

Knees to Chest (Pavanmuktasana)

Benefits:

Stretches lower back, increases spinal flexibility, massages internal organs, and loosens hips. Knees to Chest is essentially the same as the Standing Knee Squeeze except it is practiced in a supine position.

Instructions:

VARIATION A: KNEE TO CHEST

1. Lie on back with arms at sides.
2. Bring right knee to chest. Hold knee to chest with interlocked hands.

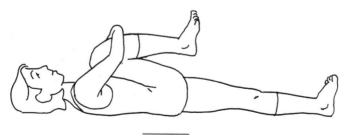

3. Keep left leg engaged and touching floor, with foot flexed upward.
4. Hold pose for three to six breaths. Repeat on opposite side. Repeat pose two to three times.
5. Come out of pose by releasing hug and lowering bent leg to floor.

VARIATION B: KNEES TO CHEST

1. Lie on back with arms at sides.
2. Bring both knees to chest.
3. Put arms around both knees in a hug, raising upper body and touching head to knees.

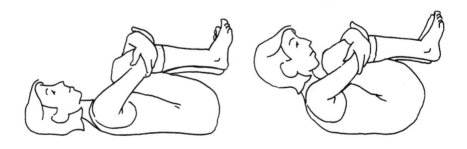

4. Hold pose for three to six breaths.
5. Come out of pose by releasing arms, placing them at sides, and extending legs back into starting position. Place head and upper back against floor. Repeat pose two to three times.

Tips:
- Relax neck and shoulders.

- This pose is good for releasing tension in the lower back and as a counterpose after backward bending poses like the Bridge (page 139), Locust (page 144), or Cobra (page 148).

- You will feel a stretch in your lower back, hips, and thighs.

Rating: I & II

Caution:
- Be careful if you have neck problems.

Lying Down Twists (Jathara Parivartanasana)

Benefits:

Stretches and loosens back, increases spinal flexibility, opens chest, and promotes relaxation.

Instructions:

1. Lie on back with legs extended and ankles together, arms outstretched at sides, perpendicular to body and palms up.
2. Bend at knees so that feet are on the floor about a foot in front of buttocks. Inhale.
3. Exhale, allowing knees to drop to the left side, keeping feet on floor.

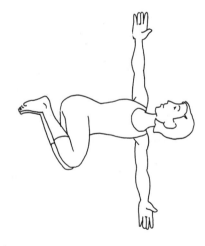

4. Turn head gently to right side. Breath three to six breaths into right side of body.

5. Inhale, returning head and legs to starting position. Repeat on opposite side. Repeat pose two to three times.

VARIATION:

1. Lie on back with legs extended and ankles together, arms outstretched at side, palms down.
2. Bend right knee, keeping right foot on floor about a foot in front of buttocks. Inhale.
3. Exhale, pressing right knee with left hand across left leg until it touches floor. Turn head to right side. Keep extended leg straight and engaged.

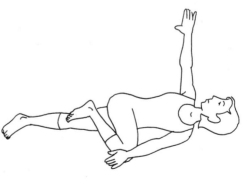

137

4. Hold pose for three to six breaths, breathing into right side of body.
5. Inhale, raising knee back to starting position.
6. Repeat on opposite side. Repeat pose two to three times.

Tips:
- Try to keep shoulders against floor.

- Keep extended leg engaged in Variation.

- You will feel a stretch in your lower and upper back, and in your hips.

Rating: I & II

Caution:
- Be careful if you have lower back problems.

Bridge (Setu Bandhasana)

Benefits:

Stretches and strengthens neck and back muscles, loosens neck and shoulders, and improves spinal flexibility. Firms legs, thighs, hips, and abdomen.

Instructions:

1. Lie on your back with bent knees, heels close to buttocks, and arms at your sides.

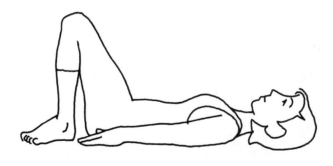

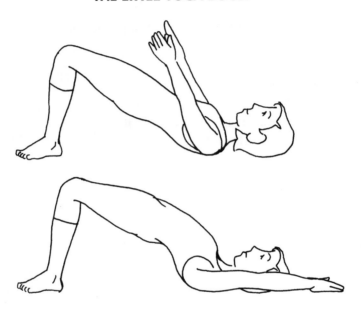

2. As you inhale, lift buttocks off the ground and slowly raise back from the floor, rolling up to upper back and shoulders, while raising your arms.

3. Continue until your arms are over your head and resting against the floor. You will feel your chin lower toward your chest as the back of your neck lengthens.

4. With an exhaling breath, slowly lower your back to the ground, vertebra by vertebra, starting at the top of the spine.

5. At the same time, raise arms over head and lower them to the floor.

6. Repeat pose three to six times.

Tips:

- Keep buttocks squeezed together when raising and lowering back to floor until lower back touches floor.

- You will feel a stretch in your thighs, back, neck, and shoulders.

Rating: I & II

Cautions:

- Be careful if you have lower back problems.

- Some women do not do this pose during the heavy flow days of their periods because the backward bending and inversion reverses the direction of the menstrual flow.

Fish (Matsyasana)

Benefits:

Stretches neck and upper and middle back, expands the chest, and increases circulation to spine and brain, stimulating thyroid, parathyroid, pituitary, and pineal glands.

Instructions:

1. Lie on your back with legs extended and feet together.
2. Place hands under buttocks, palms against the floor, and slowly arch your back and neck.
3. Support yourself with bent arms as you continue to raise chest into air. Keep legs and buttocks on the floor.
4. Rest top of head against floor. Do not support weight with head or neck.
5. Hold pose for three to six breaths.
6. Slowly straighten your spine and return to resting position, using your arms to support the back. Repeat pose two to three times.

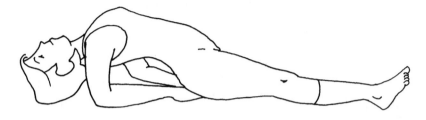

Tips:

- To modify this pose, lie on your back with your knees bent, feet flat against floor. Place a blanket or two bed pillows underneath you, perpendicular to your spine, making sure that the bulk of support is underneath your shoulder blades. Raise arms over head, resting them on the floor, palms up.

- Do not breathe too deeply; allow normal breathing.

- Keep legs together and touching floor.

- This is a good counterpose after the Bridge or Simple Inverted poses (pages 139, 154).

- Counterpose with Knees to Chest pose (page 133).

- You will feel a stretch in upper back and neck.

Rating: II

Caution: • Be careful if you have lower back problems.

Locust (Salabhasana) and Half Locust (Arhda-salabhasana)

Benefits:

Strengthens lower back, abdomen, thighs, and hips. The backward bending action aids digestion, enhances lymphatic system, stimulates adrenal glands and kidneys, and increases circulation to spine.

Instructions:

Variation A: Half Locust

1. Lie face down, chin against floor, with arms at sides, palms down.
2. Make hands into fists, thumb side against floor. Lift right leg up. Raise leg as high as you can while keeping it straight and hips on the floor. Hold pose for three breaths.
3. Slowly lower leg.
4. Repeat with left leg. Repeat pose two to three times.

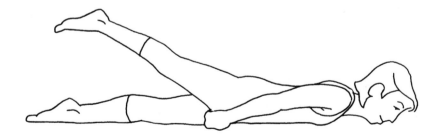

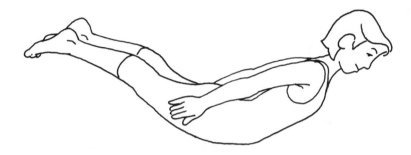

Variation B: Locust

1. Lie face down, chin against floor, with arms at sides, palms down.
2. Lift both legs up and pull arms back and away from body, raising chest and arms off of floor. Focus eyes on a point in front of you. Hold pose for three breaths.
3. Slowly lower legs and arms. Repeat pose two to three times.

Tips: • Use muscles in legs and buttocks, not lower back, to raise and lower legs.

- Relax shoulders and upper body.

- Press hip bones and pubic bone into floor to keep spine in neutral position. If it is more comfortable, you can place palms against the floor in Half Locust instead of your fists.

- Many books show these poses with the chin resting on the floor (see step 1). I prefer to place my forehead on the floor to keep my neck relaxed.

- You will feel a stretch in your back, hips, and thighs, and, with the Locust, in shoulders.

Rating: II

Cautions:

- Do not do this pose if you are pregnant.

- Be careful if you have lower back problems.

Cobra (Bhujangasana)

Benefits:

Strengthens back, abdomen, arms, and shoulders, and increases flexibility in the middle of the back. Improves oxygen intake, increases circulation to spine, and improves digestion.

Instructions:

1. Lie face down, with arms bent and tucked at sides and hands on floor at breast level, palms down. Legs and ankles should be pressed together.
2. As you inhale, slowly lift chest off of floor, using muscles in mid-back, keeping head and neck straight. Arms should not be extended or bearing weight, but tucked in and down at sides. Look straight ahead.
3. Hold pose for three to six breaths.
4. Exhale, lowering arms first, then back, one vertebra at a time from bottom of spine. Repeat pose two to three times.

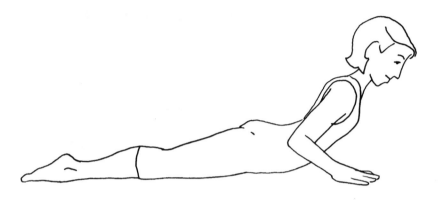

Tips:

- Keep eyes focused straight ahead.

- Keep hip bones and pubic bone pressed to floor.

- Keep shoulders down, arms tucked at sides, shoulder blades flat against back.

- Weight is not supported by arms; you should be able to lift hands off of floor and maintain pose.

- You will feel a stretch in your back, chest, shoulders, and arms.

Rating: II

Cautions:

- Be careful if you have lower back problems.

- Do not do this pose if you are pregnant.

INVERTED POSES
Plough (Halasana)

Benefits:

Stretches and strengthens hamstrings, abdomen, ankles, and feet. Relieves stiffness in shoulders and neck, and increases spinal flexibility. The forward bending action and inversion stimulate the thyroid, sex glands, liver, kidneys, and spleen.

Instructions:

1. Lie on back.
2. With arms on floor (palms down) for support, slowly lift knees to chest. Keeping knees bent, lift buttocks and roll over head, extending bent legs, until toes are touching (or pointing behind you) the floor behind the head.
3. Hold pose for several seconds or up to two minutes. Do not try to breathe deeply in this pose. Allow normal breathing, although it may be shorter and shallower.
4. Come out of pose by bringing knees to chest and slowly rolling back into a supine position, vertebra by vertebra, with arms against floor for support.

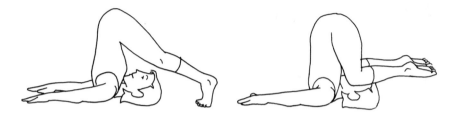

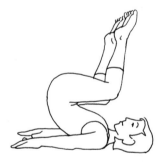

Tips:

- If it is comfortable, you can extend your legs straight in step 2.

- Lift and bend from hips, not middle of back.

- If you can't touch floor with toes, put a chair behind you and rest toes on chair.

- You will not be able to breathe normally in this position, so breathe softly.

- You will feel a stretch in back of neck, back of legs, and back.

Rating: II

Cautions:

- Be very careful with your back in this pose, especially if you have any upper back or neck tension or injuries.

- This pose puts a lot of pressure on the heart, so remember to breathe softly and relax.

- Not recommended during pregnancy.

Simple Inverted
(Viparita Karani)

Benefits:

Helps reverse the influence of gravity on internal organs. Increases circulation, strengthens the back and abdomen, and stimulates the thyroid and endocrine glands.

Instructions:

1. Lie on back.
2. Using arms to support the back, raise legs and buttocks into the air.
3. Arms will be against floor and palms holding lower back.
4. Hold pose for up to three minutes, breathing slowly.
5. Come out of pose gently and slowly. (See instructions for Plough on page 151). Bend knees to chest, place arms straight behind you, palms down. Slowly lower back to floor from top of spine, vertebra by vertebra, until buttocks touch floor. Keep head on floor.
6. Extend legs and rest for two to three minutes, breathing normally.

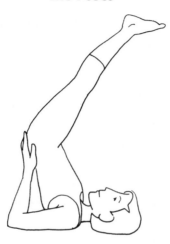

Tips:
- Keep legs and ankles together and legs straight.

- Legs and body will not be in a straight line. Body will be bent at hips with legs slightly forward, forming an approximate 120° angle with the body.

- Use the Bridge pose as a counterpose (page 139).

- You will feel a stretch in your upper back and neck.

Rating: II

Cautions:

- Do not do this pose until you have been instructed by a trained teacher. The inversion puts pressure on the heart, and may create pressure in your ears and eyes, so breathing should be soft.

- Be careful with neck and head.

- If you have any type of heart or neck problems, or high blood pressure, consult your doctor before trying this pose. Some women do not do this pose during the heavy flow days of their periods because the inversion reverses the direction of the menstrual flow.

- Not recommended during pregnancy.

RELAXING POSES

Child's Pose

Benefits:

Relaxes lower back and neck, regulates circulation, and reduces fatigue and tension.

Instructions:

1. In a kneeling position, sit on heels.
2. Lower chest to thighs, then forehead to ground, using arms to support weight as you go down.
3. Rest arms on floor, lying along legs, palms up. Hold pose for three to six breaths.

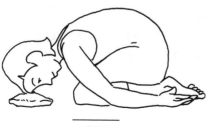

Tips:
- You can rest your forehead on a small pillow if it's more comfortable for you.

- A good relaxing pose to do in between poses and after back bends.

Rating: I & II

Relaxing Pose
(Savasana)

This pose is also called the Sponge or the Corpse. It should be done at the end of every yoga practice for at least five minutes.

Benefits:

Allows circulation and breathing to return to normal, and the mind to relax and meditate.

Instructions:

1. Lie on back with legs extended, ankles a few inches apart, and feet relaxed and falling to the side.
2. Place arms at sides and slightly away from body, palms up.
3. Relax facial muscles, neck, shoulders, arms, and legs until you feel calm and loose. Allow your breathing to return to normal flow.

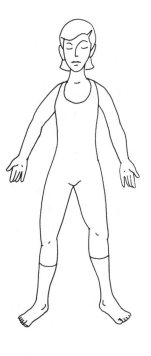

Tips:

• You may want to listen to a relaxation tape while in this pose, and cover yourself with a blanket to stay warm.

• You can use a small pillow under the backs of your knees.

Rating: I

SERIES POSES

Sun Salute (Surya Namaskar)

The Sun Salute, a series of twelve separate poses done slowly and rhythmically in coordination with the breath, is one of the most dynamic yoga exercises.

Benefits:

Stretches and strengthens all major muscle groups, increases circulation throughout the body, massages internal organs, and reduces fatigue and tension.

Instructions:

1. In a standing pose, place palms together in front of chest, breathing normally.
2. Inhale, raising chest and slowly raising arms above head, releasing palms and pointing fingertips up and behind you, lengthening the spine in a gentle stretch.

3. Exhale, bending forward from the hips and placing hands on the floor on the sides of each foot. Place your forehead as close to your knees as possible, keeping your legs straight. (You can bend your knees slightly if you need to. See Standing Forward Bend, page 92.)

4. Inhale as you push your right leg back behind your body, bending the left leg and supporting yourself with your hands. You will end up in a lunge position, with your hands and right knee touching the floor. Hold your body upright and tall, looking straight ahead.

5. Exhale, raising your right knee off of the floor and pushing your left leg back behind your body until you are in a push-up position. Hold your breath while keeping back and head in a straight line. Look down toward the floor. Inhale.

6. Exhale, bending your knees to the floor and touching your chest and chin to the floor, keeping your hips raised.

7. Inhale, raising chest off of floor, sliding chest through extended arms. Keep elbows tucked against the sides of your body, and keep shoulders down and away from ears. (This is similar to the Cobra pose, but with the arms extended. If it is more comfortable for you, keep your arms bent in this step. Be careful not to strain your lower back.) Look straight ahead.

8. Exhale, putting weight into arms and curling your toes against the floor. Raise hips into the air to form an inverted "V" as in Downward Facing Dog pose. Arms and legs should be straight, feet should be flat against floor. (You may only be able to keep toes on floor, that's okay.) Keep your shoulders back and down from ears.

9. Inhale, pulling right foot to the front of body and aligning it between hands, leaving left leg extended behind you with left knee touching the floor.

10. Exhale, pulling left foot to the front of body, ending in a standing forward bend with hands touching floor on sides of feet.

11. Inhale, rolling body slowly from hips, vertebra by vertebra, into a standing position. As you raise your chest, extend your arms over your head, reaching your fingertips up and behind you, lengthening the spine in a gentle stretch.

12. Exhale, returning to original position. Repeat series, switching leg positions in step 4 and in step 9, (i.e., extending the opposite leg than in the first round in each step.) Repeat series two to ten times.

Tips:
- The Sun Salute series is difficult to master. This exercise can be hard on your lower back, so take your time, and don't push yourself too hard. Ask your teacher to show you how to coordinate your movements with your breath and how to protect your back during this exercise.

- The Sun Salute can be done first thing in the morning after warm-up exercises.

- You will feel a stretch in all major muscle groups.

- Counterpose the Sun Salute with Relaxing pose.

Rating: II

Cautions:
- Be careful if you have back problems, high blood pressure, or dizziness.

- If you are pregnant, consult your doctor before practicing this series.

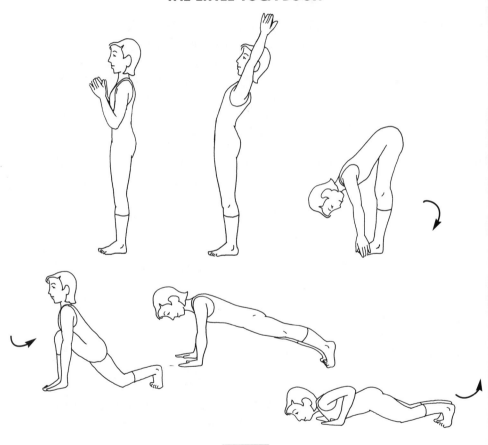

The Poses

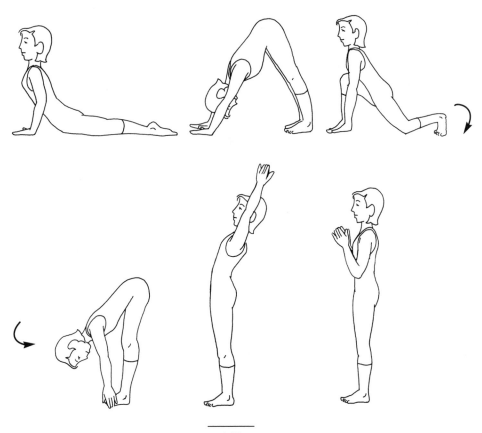

165

7/Sample Workouts

The workouts listed below will get you started in your daily practice. As you learn more exercises in class you can make up your own routines with your favorite poses.

Before you begin a workout, spend a few minutes on breathing and warm-up exercises. Remember to rest for a minute or two between each pose. These workouts and the times are merely guidelines. Depending on how long you warm up and how many rounds of each pose you do, you might take more or less time than suggested. Don't worry if you can't finish all the poses in the time given; go at your own pace.

5–10 minute practice
Breathing exercises
Warm-ups

10–15 minute practice
Breathing exercises
Warm-ups
Mountain
Half Moon
Cat
Spinal Twist
Knees to Chest
Relaxing

10–15 minute practice
Breathing exercises
Warm-ups
Sun Salute (repeat six times)
Relaxing

10–15 minute practice
Breathing exercises

Warm-ups
Cat
Knee to Chest
Lying Down Twist
Head to Knee
Downward Facing Dog
Child's
Relaxing

10–15 minute practice
Breathing exercises
Warm-ups
Half Moon
Triangle
Head to Knee
Spinal Twist
Bridge
Child's
Relaxing

15–20 minute practice
Breathing exercises

Warm-ups
Dancer
Tree
Cat
Cobra
Child's
Butterfly
Side Bend Over Legs
Lying Down Twist
Bridge
Knees to Chest
Relaxing

20–30 minute practice
Breathing exercises
Warm-ups
Warrior
Eagle
Downward Facing Dog
Kneeling Chest Expander
Cowhead
Head to Knee

Spinal Twist
Locust or Half Locust
Cobra
Child's
Simple Inverted
Fish
Knees to Chest
Relaxing

20–30 minute practice
Breathing exercises
Warm-ups
Dancer
Eagle
Standing Forward Bend
Butterfly
Spinal Twist
Side Bend Over Legs
Cowhead
Cat
Downward Facing Dog

Leg Lifts
Lying Down Twists
Locust
Child's
Simple Inverted
Relaxing

30–40 minute practice
Breathing exercises
Warm-ups
Half Moon
Triangle
Standing Forward Bend
Seated Arm Stretch
Downward Facing Dog
Foot Stretch
Head to Knee
Lying Down Twist
Cobra
Child's

Locust
Child's
Plough
Knees to Chest
Relaxing

30–40 minute practice
Breathing exercises
Warm-ups
Standing Knee Squeeze
Standing Forward Bend
Seated Arm Stretch
Spinal Twist
Pigeon
Child's
Cat
Leg Lifts
Bridge
Knees to Chest
Simple Inverted
Relaxing

YOGA ACTIVITY AND SPORTS CHART

A well-rounded yoga routine can prepare you for sports, prevent injuries, and even enhance your performance by improving your strength, flexibility, and balance. The chart below lists in alphabetical order several poses that are beneficial in conditioning your body for different sports and activities. The poses can be done before and after activity.

Breathing exercises can be done before all activities, and relaxing poses (Child's, Relaxing) can be done after all activities.

Activity/Sport   Poses

Computer use   Arm Reach, Arm Stretch, Bridge, Cat, Cowhead, Downward Facing Dog, Eagle, Head to Knee, Kneeling Chest Expander, Neck Stretch, Seated Arm Stretch, Shoulder Roll, Spinal Twist, Warrior.

Gardening   Arm Stretch, Cat, Child's, Cowhead, Foot Stretch, Half Moon, Head to Knee, Lying Down Twists, Neck Stretch, Plough, Seated Arm Stretch, Shoulder Roll, Triangle.

Sitting at a desk Arm Reach*, Bridge, Cat, Dancer, Downward Facing Dog, Eagle, Fish, Half Moon, Head to Knee, Knees to Chest, Leg Lifts, Lying Down Twists, Mountain, Neck Stretch*, Relaxing, Seated Forward Bend, Shoulder Roll*, Spinal Twist, Tree, Triangle, Warrior. (*Several of these poses, or variations, can be done while sitting at a desk. Also see Computer use, and poses for Poor Posture, page 182).

Basketball Cowhead, Dancer, Downward Facing Dog, Kneeling Chest Expander, Lying Down Twists, Shoulder Roll, Standing Forward Bend, Standing Knee Squeeze, Warrior.

Baseball/Softball Arm Reach, Cat, Cowhead, Half Moon, Kneeling Chest Expander, Pigeon, Standing Forward Bend, Tree.

Bicycling Dancer, Kneeling Chest Expander, Knees to Chest, Neck Stretch, Seated Forward Bend, Spinal Twist.

Cross-country Skiing

Butterfly, Cobra, Dancer, Half Moon, Pigeon, Standing Forward Bend, Triangle.

Dancing Cat, Dancer, Downward Facing Dog, Foot Stretch, Head to Knee, Leg Lifts, Lying Down Twists, Standing Knee Squeeze, Tree, Triangle.

Downhill Skiing Butterfly, Cat, Pigeon, Side Bend Over Legs, Spinal Twist, Standing Forward Bend, Warrior.

Golf Arm Stretch, Bridge, Cowhead, Downward Facing Dog, Eagle, Half Moon, Lying Down Twists, Neck Stretch, Shoulder Roll, Triangle.

Hiking/Mountaineering

Bridge, Downward Facing Dog, Foot Stretch, Knees to Chest, Standing Forward Bend, Triangle.

Kayaking/Canoeing

Arm Stretch, Bridge, Child's, Cobra, Half Moon, Kneeling Chest Expander, Seated Forward Bend, Spinal Twist, Warrior.

Running/Walking

Bridge, Butterfly, Cat, Dancer, Foot Stretch, Half Moon, Head to Knee, Pigeon, Triangle, Warrior.

Skating

Cat, Foot Stretch, Half Moon, Standing Knee Squeeze, Triangle.

Soccer

Bridge, Butterfly, Downward Facing Dog, Neck Stretch, Pigeon, Side Bend Over Legs, Triangle.

Swimming

Arm Stretch, Cobra, Cowhead, Downward Facing Dog, Kneeling Chest Expander, Knees to Chest, Plough, Spinal Twist.

Tennis   Butterfly, Cowhead, Dancer, Eagle, Half Moon, Head to Knee, Spinal Twist, Standing Knee Squeeze, Warrior.

Yoga Body Part Chart

If you want to exercise specific areas of the body, the chart below will help you reference the appropriate poses in this book.

Area	Pose
Abdomen	Bridge, Cobra, Half Moon, Leg Lifts, Locust and Half Locust, Mountain, Plough, Simple Inverted.
Ankles	Downward Facing Dog, Eagle, Foot Stretch, Plough, Tree, Triangle, Thunderbolt.
Arms	Arm Reach, Arm Stretch, Cat, Cobra, Downward Facing Dog, Seated Arm Stretch.

Back	Bridge, Cat, Child's, Cobra, Downward Facing Dog, Eagle, Fish, Half Moon, Head to Knee, Kneeling Chest Expander, Knees to Chest, Leg Lifts, Locust and Half Locust, Lying Down Twists, Plough, Seated Arm Stretch, Seated Forward Bend, Simple Inverted, Spinal Twist, Standing Forward Bend, Standing Knee Squeeze, Warrior.
Balance	Cat Variation, Dancer, Eagle, Mountain, Standing Knee Squeeze, Tree, Triangle, Warrior.
Chest	Cobra, Downward Facing Dog, Fish, Kneeling Chest Expander, Lying Down Twists, Pigeon, Triangle, Warrior.
Feet	Dancer, Foot Stretch, Half Moon, Standing Knee Squeeze, Tree, Triangle.
Hands/Wrists	Arm Stretch, Cat, Cobra, Seated Arm Stretch.

Hips	Bridge, Butterfly, Cat Variation, Dancer, Eagle, Half Moon, Knees to Chest, Locust and Half Locust, Pigeon, Side Bend Over Legs, Standing Knee Squeeze, Spinal Twist, Tree, Triangle, Warrior.
Legs	Bridge, Butterfly, Dancer, Downward Facing Dog, Eagle, Half Moon, Head to Knee, Leg Lifts, Locust and Half Locust, Mountain, Plough, Seated Forward Bend, Side Bend Over Legs, Standing Forward Bend, Standing Knee Squeeze, Thunderbolt, Tree, Triangle, Warrior.
Knees	Head to Knee, Thunderbolt, Warrior.
Neck	Bridge, Cat, Child's, Cobra, Fish, Neck Stretch, Plough, Simple Inverted.
Shoulders	Arm Reach, Bridge, Cat Variation, Cobra, Cowhead, Eagle, Kneeling Chest Expander, Plough, Seated Arm Stretch, Shoulder Roll, Simple Inverted, Warrior.

Sides of Torso Half Moon, Side Bend Over Legs, Triangle.

Spinal Flexibility Bridge, Cat, Cobra, Half Moon, Knees to Chest, Lying Down Twists, Spinal Twist, Triangle.

YOGA HEALTH CHART

Yoga poses can be good supplements to traditional health treatments because they relax the body, calm the mind, and improve respiration and circulation. By slowing down, focusing on your breathing, and stretching your body, you can reduce tension and help the healing process.

Different yoga teachers may have varying opinions about which poses are most beneficial for specific conditions. Because the poses suggested here come from a handful of different sources, I have listed several poses for each condition to allow you more flexibility in your practice.

Please remember that you should consult a doctor if you are sick or in pain, and yoga should never be a substitute for medical care. Your doctor and yoga teacher can help you find the poses that best suit your health needs.

Health Conditions	Pose
Anxiety	Breathing exercises, Cat, Child's, Head to Knee, Knees to Chest, Lying Down Twists, Relaxing, Spinal Twist, Standing and Seated Forward Bends, Standing Knee Squeeze.
Arthritis	Arm Reach, Breathing exercises, Bridge, Cat, Cobra, Cowhead, Head to Knee, Mountain, Plough, Relaxing, Seated Arm Stretch, Simple Inverted, Spinal Twist.
Asthma	Arm Reach, Breathing exercises, Bridge, Dancer, Fish, Knee to Chest, Locust, Mountain, Relaxing.
Backache	Breathing exercises, Bridge, Cat, Cobra, Cowhead, Downward Facing Dog, Fish,

Head to Knee, Knees to Chest, Kneeling Chest Expander, Lying Down Twists, Plough, Spinal Twist, Standing Forward Bend.

Constipation

Breathing exercises, Cat, Cobra, Fish, Half Moon, Head to Knee, Kneeling Chest Expander, Knees to Chest, Lying Down Twists, Spinal Twist, Standing and Seated Forward Bends, Standing Knee Squeeze, Sun Salute.

Depression

Breathing exercises, Cobra, Dancer, Knees to Chest, Plough, Simple Inverted, Spinal Twist, Tree, Triangle.

Fatigue

Breathing exercises, Bridge, Child's, Cobra, Downward Facing Dog, Locust, Neck Stretch, Plough, Relaxing, Simple Inverted, Sun Salute.

Headache	Breathing exercises, Cat, Cobra, Lying Down Twists, Neck Stretch, Plough, Relaxing, Simple Inverted, Spinal Twist.
Hemorrhoids	Fish, Plough, Simple Inverted.
Indigestion	Cat, Cobra, Half Moon, Mountain, Plough, Relaxing, Standing Knee Squeeze, Spinal Twist.
Insomnia	Alternate Nostril Breathing exercise, Complete Breath exercise, Cat, Child's, Fish, Neck Stretch, Plough, Relaxing, Simple Inverted.
Menopause	Cat, Cobra, Downward Facing Dog, Fish, Plough, Relaxing, Simple Inverted, Warrior.
Nervousness/Tension	Alternate Nostril Breathing exercise, Child's, Half Moon, Mountain, Relaxing, Simple Inverted, Thunderbolt, Warrior.

PMS	Breathing exercises, Bridge, Cat, Cobra, Lying Down Twists, Pigeon, Relaxing, Simple Inverted.
Poor Posture	Cobra, Cowhead, Mountain, Tree, Triangle. (All poses that strengthen the abdominal muscles, loosen the shoulder area, and stretch back and neck muscles.)
Varicose Veins	Plough, Simple Inverted.

Index

Index

Index

Index

Index

Index